T0128837

TOOTH SENSE

TOOTH SENSE

UNCOVERING HIDDEN SECRETS OF BETTER DENTISTRY AND LIVING

Why do patients respond so differently to essentially the same procedure?

JEFFREY A. ORAS, DMD

iUniverse, Inc.
Bloomington

Tooth Sense
Uncovering Hidden Secrets of Better Dentistry and Living

iUniverse books may be ordered through booksellers or by contacting:

iUniverse
1663 Liberty Drive
Bloomington, IN 47403
www.iuniverse.com
1-800-Authors (1-800-288-4677)

ISBN: 978-1-4759-6532-2 (sc)
ISBN: 978-1-4759-6534-6 (hc)
ISBN: 978-1-4759-6533-9 (e)

Library of Congress Control Number: 2012922828

Printed in the United States of America

iUniverse rev. date: 12/17/2012

To my wife, Marie, and my parents, Andrew and Margaret. You have taught me more than I could have hoped for.

To my patients who have propelled me to continue to be better. Thank you!

CONTENTS

Acknowledgments

There are many people who have influenced, supported, and challenged me along my journey. I am grateful for all teaching I have received and the examples I have found not just useful but inspiring. Very often I was not aware of their value at the time.

First and utmost, I would like to thank my wife, Marie, who has patiently allowed me the time to devote countless hours to this project. Also, I thank my parents, Andrew and Margaret Oras. It is said that every family is a complex culture unto itself, each family story a unique and complex expression of the quest for love, support, and connection, a quest full of successes and errors. My story is no exception. Out of the satisfactions and pains of my life in my family growing up, I am grateful for acquiring a heritage of curiosity and capacity for self-knowledge and wider vision, as well as an ultimate sense of confidence and compassion. That being said, this book would not have been possible without your sacrifice and support that allowed me the tremendous opportunity to pursue and experience the satisfaction of a career in dentistry.

My writing coach Bruce Bergquist was able to help me simplify, clarify, and organize. He and his wife, Betsy Bergquist, helped me hone the concepts in *Tooth Sense*. I have been informed in many subtle ways by their teaching and coaching of the skills and processes of relationship-building developed by Harville Hendrix, PhD, and Helen LaKelly Hunt, PhD, and known as the Couples Dialogue.

I would also like to thank my staff: Beverly Ricci, Jean Evers, Ashley Morin, and Kristen Belcastro. They have endured my travails and enriched my understanding through the ongoing process of developing my ideas. Without their support, this book would not have been possible.

Over the years I have been fortunate to benefit from many teachers who expanded my vision of dentistry far beyond what I acquired in professional training. I would like especially to recognize Susan Coakley, Janet Straightarrow, and Steven Cuoco for their dedication as healers in helping me see past what I have called the "missed cues" of my earlier life. They have helped me see how intuition, empathy, and compassion may be applied to dentistry as well as to all dimensions of personal consciousness. I believe I am more open and authentic because of their wisdom.

I'd also like to thank Patricia Garvey. She has been my muse while writing this book. Her active listening made this experience a major growth experience in my life.

There have been many patients whose personal sharing with me has impelled me to be more precise in conceptualizing aspects of what I have come to term "tooth sense." There are too many to list them all. However, one patient stands out. Cathy E. Stoops-McFarlane has helped me clarify and expand much of my image of the oral cavity as not simply a collection of hard and soft tissue but also a geographical quilt of life experience.

I need to acknowledge the influence of Dietrich Klinghardt, MD, an integrative physician with whom I have studied. I was fortunate to find him in my quest for the right practice model, one that included both traditional and holistic components. He helped transform my perspective and helped me see that healing takes place in realms other than the physical and that the heart of effective treatment may involve accessing the emotional and other levels of experience. Dr. Klinghardt identifies five distinct levels as the basis of his teaching. I've included a link to a chart of these levels in the resources section.

Ralph Wilson, ND, is an extremely knowledgeable practitioner whom I met while studying with Dr. Klinghardt. He has charted precise neurological links between teeth and our other organs, and the emotional and other correspondences. This chart is included in the illustrations section.

Sinikka Laine, another patient, is responsible for the front cover artwork. *Oneness*, a painting done originally in 1997 as a way of paying homage to her father, seemed an especially appropriate way of further recognizing my late father. Its main color, indigo, is associated with the hypothalamus and pituitary glands, whose proper functions are essential to the health of teeth. Both this color and the overall balance and design of the piece convey a sense of healing and unity of all of life. Apart from her artwork, Sinikka's wisdom and wide vision have also broadened my perspectives in many ways.

Finally, I would especially like to thank my many patients who have given me their trust and who have stretched to allow themselves to be vulnerable at the same time. I consider them all valued companions on the journey. Meaningful life work is always based on compassionate and empathic relationships. Dentistry is no exception. Neither is the ongoing common quest for all of us to find our own individual tooth sense.

Introduction—
In Pursuit of Tooth Sense

Who hasn't taken a seat in the dental chair without some sense of foreboding about what is coming next? At such moments, thoughts and feelings ranging in intensity from simple concern to mild anxiety to flat-out fear and dread might be coursing through you. Chances are you know what I am talking about.

Whatever the intensity of your thoughts or feelings in such moments, your reactions are perfectly understandable, appropriate, and essential. They are also widely misunderstood, misjudged, and mistreated. You do not have a character defect or lack of willpower.

Whatever your response to dentistry has been in the past, *Tooth Sense* is about helping you demystify the sources of the fear and misunderstanding. It is about replacing your fears and misunderstandings with a new perspective that can help you feel safe and confident—not just in dentistry, but in the way you view it and experience it. Think of it as a working guide toward reclaiming your power while in the chair.

This power has long remained mostly hidden from view for patients, even from the dental profession itself, in terms of how dentists deliver care. Our general operational modes involve ignoring, sedating, or suppressing our patients' anxieties. Without intending to do so, we have left the underlying fears unprocessed, perpetuated, and even magnified.

I have long found this phenomenon troubling. My dissatisfaction fueled my motivation to stay with my quest—and now to share it freely, incomplete as it may be. The good news is that I came to see that my understanding, though the result of following many false leads and though full of personal doubt, really could and would distill into some simple, rich, and self-empowering "tattoos" for my patients and for me.

It is ironic that a key to understanding and demystifying dental anxieties and fears is held within anatomical structures right inside the mouth. These structures create a vulnerability that humans have had to adjust to for forty thousand years.

My passion for exploring what is known about these structures and their anatomical subtleties, and giving them an inclusive name, led to my coining the term "tooth sense" as a way of referring to the numerous complex activities and functions of teeth and the oral region. The term refers variously to

- how teeth sense (or in some ways don't sense), and the significance of this selectivity;
- how teeth act as modulators of our life experiences;
- how an anatomical feature in the mouth contributes to a unique vulnerability that all humans experience;
- how this vulnerability manifests differently in each of us;
- how each of us manifests this innate vulnerability—not only in the dental chair but in life.

My quest has been personal as well as professional. Even though I didn't realize it at the time, this quest began very early in life—in fact, years before the thought of becoming a dentist would even cross my mind.

It began as complex confusion about the behavior, thoughts, and feelings I observed and experienced growing up in central New Jersey. From my earliest years, I was a close and sensitive observer. Early on, I had an intense motivation and curiosity about why people, including myself, thought, felt, and acted in ways that they did. I saw all of us continuously responding to situations in ways that often made no sense—and did not seem to serve anyone. I was thinking big, at least as big as I could, and I was trying to sort things out.

Then, of course, I had few clues. As a nine-year-old, for instance, I didn't know exactly what questions to ask, let alone what the answers might be. I lacked the language and the confidence to use it, even if I had such language. I was simply dissatisfied. I had a vague, big vision that life could be better. The stories of my early life that comprise the first three chapters by no means constitute an autobiography. I've selected these vignettes because they give an inside look at a few of my most significant early experiences and thoughts.

My formal education up through much of college did not inspire me or seem relevant to the workings of my mind and imagination. It was what had to be done to get the ticket to the next step, even if I had no career in mind. But the conflicting second impulse was also at work—the impulse to break out of the mold, to challenge what were acceptable life choices and behaviors and ask more of life and how I might best fulfill mine.

This ambivalence has still not been fully resolved. It has driven me over much of the thirty years since I began my life in dentistry. It was with me as a science major in college, then as a part-time chair-side dental assistant, a dental student, a young dentist in a large established practice, and, during the last twenty years, in my own active practice. On one hand, I have embraced and developed all the elements of a successful conventional practice. On the other hand, as

I went about my daily business of treating patients over the years, a simple question always provoked me deeply: Why do patients seem to respond so differently to essentially the same procedure? I could never dismiss my concerns with a shrug. *People are all just different. That is the way it is. Just deal with it.*

This dissatisfaction has been the driver that has transformed my practice and my approach to it. What I have learned has impelled respect, compassion, and empathy for what the patient is dealing with. It has also helped me frame my own work with more compassion. I have become easier on myself, and less of a perfectionist, as I juggle technical challenges or a taxing daily schedule. And perhaps paradoxically, my actual dentistry seems to have improved. I feel able to tap into my own intuition better so that I can sense, and connect to, what patients are feeling so that I can offer them even more comfort and ease.

My insight has allowed me to shift my attention from my earlier coping methods of not only fixing the tooth but also trying to "fix" the patient as well. I instead have found myself seeing things more clearly, understanding that any physical sign of discomfort, any apparent resistance during the dental-care process, is not truly a problem, just something that has come up and is offering a clue as to what is beneath. I can breathe more easily and work more naturally with the understanding that any problems that arise during the diagnostic, treatment, planning, scheduling, delivery, or maintenance phases are influenced by "tooth sense."

I do not wish to disparage the evolved and evolving state of dental technology. The years prior to my entry into the profession, roughly beginning at the end of World War II, and continuing to the present, modern dentistry has seen remarkable advances in providing care. Much disease and suffering has been ameliorated. The incidence of infection has been greatly reduced. The quality of patients' lives in terms of ability to chew, to speak properly, and to look and feel good about themselves has been very much enhanced. Most importantly, procedures have come to be performed with much more comfort than ever before. All of these improvements have done nothing less than transform the standard of care available today.

When I graduated from dental school in 1987, this standard of care was expanding in the form of new dental equipment and improved materials, techniques, and methods of care. It was natural that I got caught up in this technological wave in dental school, dutifully striving to be proficient in my new career. Once I was out in the world, my focus was not entirely misplaced; I would have found it difficult not to include these features in my practice.

Yet buying into this emerging way of doing things was no substitute for following a yet-to-be-formed wider vision of care. I could not escape a nagging awareness that dentistry is work commonly filled with emotional charge for patients, despite the dentist's suppression of pain, which was the dominant mode of care. In fact, the suppression in some ways magnified the emotional charge since it remained unprocessed. And perhaps most significant of all, the emotional charge for patients was not restricted to the 5–10 percent of the population that could be "diagnosed" as dental phobic; it was present to one degree or another in everyone. It was part of what makes us all human. From then on, I could never look at my work as simply, or even primarily, technical. Dental treatment was work involving a human team of providers and patients, and the business was at least as much about communication and connection as it was about restoring a filling or extracting a tooth.

So *Tooth Sense* is not simply for the anxious or phobic; it is for anyone curious about what happens when patients enter the dentist's office for treatment, regardless of how adept they may be at presenting themselves. It proposes insights that have as much to do with everyday people who need simple, straightforward dental care as they do for the severely challenged. Though somewhat technical in places, the information presented is not taken from dental school textbooks. It is not concerned with pharmaceuticals or bright, shiny gadgets you can buy when you have finished reading. Instead it addresses larger scientific and nonscientific questions about the subtle physical and neurological workings of that part of the human anatomy and physiology whose territory I enter every day—not just the teeth but also the connected and associated structures within the mouth, tongue, larynx, throat, and the swallowing manager known as the epiglottis.

It is as if these structures hold the key for whether the person will respond with ease or—if there is strain or tension—how that strain or tension will physically and emotionally manifest itself. It is as if the teeth themselves working together with other structures in the mouth are themselves the modulators of experience. Ironically, all this operation is hidden from view from patients themselves.

Some of what I have delved into is well accepted; some is more theoretical and speculative. I have been very constructively challenged to make this material user-friendly (and even interesting!) to the nonscientist while staying accurate and not dumbing it down. If, despite my efforts, you find some material daunting, especially the content of chapters 6 and 8, please feel free to pass them by and move on. The rest of the book can still speak its essence to you.

For the most part, I have proceeded chronologically so that you can not only experience what I am sharing as it unfolded, but also so you might have a greater awareness of how my growth and life experiences have shaped this quest. The first three chapters explore, describe, and reflect upon my early life, growing up in central New Jersey, in my family, in my neighborhood, and in America in the 1960s and '70s, prior to my even considering dentistry as a career. They describe in detail a few landmark experiences that have stuck with me.

Chapters 4 through 11 follow my quest to create a practice that met the needs of both patients and me, personally as well as professionally. Where I have referred to specific situations, I have changed the names of the patients involved.

While I make scientific citations and describe the pieces I found deeply relevant to my quest, *Tooth Sense* is a narrative, not a piece awaiting peer review. The book is not footnoted, and there is no bibliography. It is designed to be understood by readers with a curiosity about the topics—but without a special scientific background. I have included a references section, but have not followed academic citation format to the letter. Many of my references are to articles, monographs, and websites. More information about my references to specific works, or names of authors or practitioners, is in almost all cases available through a basic keyword Internet search, should you wish to take a deeper look for yourself. These are not obscure references. I have included a few illustrations where they served to explain better than words.

Tooth Sense concludes with what might be called a status report. While pursuing the areas covered here, I have also had in mind a number of other fields of study whose further exploration might shed light on the unique activity that I call "tooth sense." These fields include biology, psychology, sociology, anthropology, gender studies, and Chinese medicine. I'm also interested in the evolutionary aspects of genetics and society. True to my nature, I have not ruled out anything as being insufficiently scientific or even not scientific at all. I have a special interest in further exploration of the role of hormones as the modulators of the transmission of energy from one part of the body to another. There is much to be found by researching the richly developing field of neuroscience. I end with a brief summary of each of these as a to-do list for the future.

Perhaps a further disclaimer is in order. *Tooth Sense* is about unfolding new understandings and building a tentative case for the very existence of "tooth sense" while acknowledging that it is not "proving" anything. In fact, the healthy perspective for me is that our knowledge of the human brain, the human nervous system, and how we all behave, think, and feel is still very primitive. I've heard that the three pounds of "gray matter" that make up the human brain is more complex in its structure and function than the external physical universe itself. So this journey is not likely to be ending soon. If it is about "proving" anything, it is perhaps about validating the satisfaction that one person can achieve by holding on to and pursuing a vision and the possibility to improving life for oneself and others. As the maxim goes, "Life is a journey, not a destination."

And finally, as I will be reiterating in my final chapter, it also comes with an invitation to those motivated to join the conversation on this emerging understanding. My dental practice is ultimately based on creating and supporting meaningful relationships with patients. I would gladly do the same with interested readers. Perhaps this book will prompt some potential collaborators to join me in my evolving quest to more fully grasp "tooth sense."

1

MORE THAN FINDING THE WALLET

Long before I knew anything about the profession, the path to my career in dentistry was being set. The circumstances of my family, my neighborhood, the state of our country in the 1970s, and my own personal brand of curiosity, reflection, genetics, and the imprint of experience were setting my psychological and emotional table.

I've found myself later in life revisiting some specific memories and creating a small journal of vignettes that capture some "Kodak moments." I'm including several of these vignettes in this chapter and the two that follow, in order to shed light on who I am, how I chose dentistry as my profession, how I came to pursue my own path, and how I came to write this book.

In June 1971, my family took a vacation in the White Mountains of New Hampshire. One morning, not long after my parents, my younger sister, and I had driven away from the small motel where we had stayed the previous night, a crisis arose. My father couldn't find his wallet. The last time he had seen it was while packing the car.

A lost wallet is always a concern. For my father, it was cause for high anxiety. He pulled the car over to the side of the highway, and while fumbling feverishly through the glove box, his pockets, and everything within arm's reach, he boomed orders for everyone to be quiet. This order was unnecessary. The rest of us were already frozen as statues.

My mother and sister, sighing in unison, seemed to say without saying anything, "Oh boy. What now?"

The air seemed to have gone out of their bodies as if they were balloons. The smiles that had radiated from their faces deflated in anxious frowns, and what had been my sister's bouncing up and down gave way to almost mirroring my father's body language. Her whole body stiffened against the backrest.

Meanwhile, my father stared straight ahead, his hands squeezing the steering wheel, his body stiff. Noticing a part of his face in the rearview mirror, I caught a blank fixed stare. It was a familiar scenario. I was not new to seeing him this way. It was how my father reacted when he was not in control or when people around him were not doing what they were supposed to do—even though he had not indicated what they were supposed to be doing. Dad was angry, and the rest of us were in hiding.

But I was about to break the script for this scene. I was about to take my cue from a newfound place.

The previous day, I had caught my first fish. It was just a trout, but I was nine years old; to me, it could have been a marlin. This crisis had interrupted a pleasant mental trout reverie—the nibble on the line, the tug on the line, the give-and-take with the energy on the other end, my gradual taking charge of this transaction, the shiny fish appearing below the surface and then splashing into daylight as I lifted it dangling to a grassy spot on the shore. It wasn't a keeper. So, with my father's assistance, I had unhooked it, held it firmly, and placed it back in the water. It all had taken only a short time, but it had seemed to unfold in slow motion. The experience defied any normal sense of time. Success! How much to be cherished!

Now I found myself in a state of high alert. While my mother and sister did and said nothing, I was taking it all in. During the next few moments, I prepared to do something I had never done before. It was as if the mold that held me was suddenly broken.

This instantaneous change created a rush that made my skin tingle. I was suddenly aware of everything just as much in slow motion as I had experienced landing my first fish the previous day. My mind blanked on everything except the half face I could see in the rearview mirror and shouts continuing from the driver's seat as my father continued fumbling. His showpiece Cadillac Sedan de Ville—its leather interior, dazzling dashboard, and impressive length notwithstanding—was of no comfort.

Over and above the words, I found myself saying, almost brightly, "Hey, Dad, let's go back and see if we can find it." My suggestion seemed so obvious. Yet I could see that no one else in the car had any presence of mind; it was up to me to save the day. My mother and sister were surely useless, and my father was just inconsolably confused. I was the ready one.

I was so confident in the moment that I was actually not surprised when my father took my idea and responded by immediately turning the car around and heading back to retrace our tracks. Though the road, US Route 3, was a major highway, and it was midday, I recall eeriness. The road may have been crowded, but it felt empty to me. Without any conscious thought, I leaned forward so that my arms straddled the space between the two front seats. I wanted a full view of the road ahead. I am not sure what I thought I would see. But I was in charge, even though I had in fact no conscious surveillance strategy. I was just acting on automatic pilot with total focus in response to a crisis.

I don't remember the exact distance we had traveled when he had discovered the loss. It must have been a long way from the motel. At any rate, we drove for quite a while. No one saw anything. There was talk that even if the wallet were by some remote chance on the side of the road, it would be too small to detect. I had a one-point plan: keep my eyes peeled. We were nearly all the way back to the motel, when out of the corner of my eye, just as we were passing it by, I saw something. It was almost as if I had felt it without actually seeing it. It happened in the blink of an eye.

I yelled, "Stop the car."

My father backed to where I had seen—or thought I had seen— something. Yes, there was a small rectangular object. He and I got out and as we reached it. Sure enough, his wallet was right there on the road.

Later we surmised that he had put it on the car roof, and in all of the hurried activity to get to our next destination before dark, he had forgotten about it. But in that moment, my father and I had a moment to be savored together. To say that I was proud would be an understatement. And I had never seen my father so happy. He gave me a hug, and his smile was the widest I had seen. Meanwhile, my mother and sister had remained in the rear seat as if to leave this moment to us. I looked away from my father and caught an astonished look on their faces. In the moment, they seemed a million miles away. This was a moment to be shared only with my father.

The connection that my father and I had in that moment left me feeling special in many ways. I felt special in what I accomplished, but it was more, much more. In that moment it was as if my thoughts, feelings, and beliefs all coalesced into an indelible, firm sense of myself as not just competent, but valued for that competence by my family, especially my father. Although there were no trumpets heralding this event, inside of me I just knew that I was good. I had purpose for not only myself, but for others. I had known the spot we were in and what it called for. I had been able to shine, even lead, and not only help my family avoid a huge inconvenience, but to feel confident I could help us survive other potential calamities that might befall us due to any circumstance.

The stories in the next two chapters illustrate other sides of those dynamics. This story's impact continued after leaving home and, in fact, informs me now. I have "landed many fish" and "found many wallets" in my life, and for my ability to do so I am grateful to my family—in spite of, or perhaps because of, its dysfunctions and the periodic emotional chaos. One clear gift it has supplied is the ready impulse to understand and empathize, and to be a calmer witness to patients who may be experiencing treatment as an event emotionally charged with memories and associations.

What I have come to see over time, though, is that this success story also brought with it a large message of complete self-reliance, very large expectations of myself, and a propensity to see a solution only in terms of what I alone could do. Although this perspective gave me the confidence to pursue my career and to handle any situation I might encounter while treating patients, this had a significant downside for years. I found myself driven in negative ways to take on more responsibility and to consider myself uniquely gifted, more than the situation called for or was really appropriate for the situation. Looking back, seeing myself as the last lifeline of rescue—the more critical the situation, the more heroic I fantasized myself capable of being—was not only bordering on ridiculous, but it was completely counterproductive.

Where this led will become clear as the rest of this book charts my path. Yet these stories are more than just insight into my own personal biography. The greater purpose here is to acknowledge a common theme that we all share, bearing in mind that all of us have our own path based upon some sequence of events, and our response to those events. So this book as I have said in the introduction is trying to accomplish various tasks. Within this context I am not only trying to make a case for tooth sense, I wish to awaken your own introspection for the purpose beyond just how you cope during dental care. Viewing yourself in this authentic way, with integrity and dignity for all that has transpired in your life, will come in handy later in the book.

2

A Saturday Night Family Dinner

One summer evening in 1976, our family was getting ready for our typical Saturday night dinner. It was a particularly hot evening in July. My mother and father were preparing the food for the meal. Earlier in the day, they both had been working on individual projects. My father had tended to the yard, and my mother had cleaned the inside of the house. When they were cooking, it was as if they were one. My father was preparing to barbecue steaks and bake potatoes wrapped in foil while my mother was removing fresh corn from the husks in preparation for steaming and setting out the ingredients for salad and her famous coleslaw.

Around six in the evening, the summer air still held the heat of the day. Our brick ranch home was not air conditioned, yet with all the windows and doors open, the slight breeze that moved through the house seemed to vitalize the family. This was a safe, aromatic, almost idyllic time and place. I felt my parents coming together in such moments. I could almost smell the synchronicity of the project of preparing dinner. In such moments, my father was the master of his castle, barbecuing in the backyard, using the pit that was built into the exterior wall of our home. He never said so, but he seemed to be at his best when he was providing. This was usually my favorite time to be around my family.

What was sometimes missing in such moments was a clear picture of what was expected of me. I wanted to help. I was fifteen. All of my friends did routine chores. But I hesitated, with good reason. My offers, tentative as they were, at important moments like this suddenly seemed unwanted. At these times, I thought my parents regarded me as a nuisance. In fact, I often was told that my assistance was unwelcome. I just couldn't get it right.

On this particular evening, though, I did have an assignment. I was to sort kindling from the woodpile in the yard and lay the bed of sticks for starting the fire. I brought over what I thought where appropriate ingredients. My father examined my work product. There were at least three defects: my pieces were too big, they were too wet, and they weren't positioned properly. I felt lost, alone, and defeated.

Next I went inside to see what my mother was doing. As usual, she had at least three things going on at the same time. She was very good at multitasking and had everything in its place. Like a conductor, she kept her eye simultaneously on every section of her orchestra. She was cutting the cabbage, carrots, and celery for the coleslaw while keeping a watchful eye on the corn boiling on the stove. She also had several projects going on in the oven in preparation for Sunday's lunch since we were expecting her two sisters and brother.

As I was about to offer to be her sous chef, she shooed me out of the kitchen. She said, "Go, go, go!" Even in the kitchen, I was not enough.

When preparations were complete, my parents, sister, and I were seated. The food should have been appetizing, but my feelings of inadequacy had already left me uncomfortable. Also, the smile and gait that my father had exhibited earlier were gone. I always sat to his left, and it was as if someone else had taken his place because his look had turned dark. *Did I do something else wrong?* Maybe I wasn't the reason that my father's attitude had changed. My mother was very quiet. Maybe she was the source of my father's irritation. I set aside my speculations as best I could and was ready to eat.

As we started to dig into the meal, my sister and I began a conversation about something we had seen that day on TV. We had made no more than three comments when my father interrupted and said, "Jeff, you need to be more aware of what is going on. What happened to you outside? You were making the fire pit and then you just left. You know this family depends on all of us working together. We can't tolerate this lackadaisical thinking. Where did you go?"

I mustered my best defense and said, "You didn't like how I was helping you, so I left you alone."

"That's inexcusable," he said. "Once you start something with me, I need you there to complete it! That's what I was talking to you about a couple of days ago concerning your schoolwork. You only seem to apply yourself when and if you please."

I quickly lost my appetite, yet I stayed there as was expected and tried to eat my dinner. I felt an impulse to please and protect my mother and sister so they wouldn't have to take any further brunt. Despite the hurt, a part of me seemed to be staying to make sense of all this and learn more about the dynamic that was taking shape. I was wishing that experiencing this firestorm would ultimately help me figure out how I could cope.

At that point, something started to change inside me. It was as if the disconnect between my mind and my body was widening. I don't know what changed first. Was it my mind that locked trying to follow his comments—or was it my body that just seemed to freeze? If the table had spontaneously burst into flames, I don't think I could have moved. All this tension seemed to put me in some kind of altered state. I was as if time were moving slower, not exactly what I needed. I wanted him to be done. My hearing seemed to fade, turning down the volume that was coming from my father, even as he kept going on and on. It was as if he was having a conversation with himself.

The "conversation," however, was not with himself. It was directed at me. It became simply noise, garbled by the confusion of all the cues whose decryption I felt I must be missing despite my efforts at processing. What was this all about? There was no logical explanation. Perhaps it might be the tension and negative energy that my father might have in his relationship with my mother and which was somehow being redirected toward me. I intuited only enough to complicate and confuse myself. I was angry, but was the anger at my father's confusing rant at me, or was the anger at myself and my inability to link the nonverbal tension with unwarranted verbal attention? I couldn't answer that.

The flood of different feelings devolved into a strange detachment and withdrawal, not only from the conversation, but between my mind and body as well. I don't know which was greater: the frozen state of my mind, the paralysis of my body, or my sense that both mind and body were betraying me.

Underneath there was great sadness. I remember thinking that all I wanted was for the family to be happy and enjoy this fine meal on this hot summer day. That part seemed so clear to me. Why wasn't it possible for everyone else?

As this entire swirl continued to sustain my paralysis and loss of appetite, I heard my father as if from a distance start to say something I thought might be useful. But the dreaded words were *when I was your age.*

I instantly knew what was next to follow would not be useful. It always was a diatribe in which he made references to overcoming hardship, meeting challenges, and staying alert and focused. I had only the vaguest ideas of what he was referring to. Who was this person? Was he ever fifteen; if so, when and where? What challenges and hardships? And why such passionate emphasis?

At a loss for answers, his precepts washed over me. I do not recall exactly what happened thereafter. At some point he did fall silent and got up from the table, leaving me to find my way back to this place and time. Thus the prospect of an enjoyable family dinner had ended in a way so many other family events had ended, leaving me in a state of stunned and lonely devastation.

Since then, I have followed a rich personal, emotional, and spiritual path toward insight, understanding, and healing. This path has intersected and given impetus to the trajectory of my professional life.

Of great importance has been my ability to piece together some of my father's life story, known only in the vaguest terms back then. I have never uncovered all the details, and probably never will, but I have learned enough to make it clear why I had such a maelstrom of emotion, why my parents had never been able to tell me the story that would have provided me the right cues, and why I have come in many ways to behave as I have, make the decisions I have made, and eventually write this book.

The information I have has come piecemeal from my father, my mother, and from relatives. It has not come easily. Unearthing the facts was complicated by the shroud of secrecy in which it seems so painfully but tightly held. As a fifteen-year-old, I lacked this information, an appreciation of the grip of secrecy and avoidance, and the emotions that held this in place.

In 1940, when he was fifteen, the Nazis came through his village. They took him and all of the able men to a work camp. Shortly after he landed in the work camp, he escaped with a friend. He was caught soon after, and he was sent to a political prison in Berlin. I can only imagine what my father had to cope with. I never did get all the details of his next five years. What was clear was that he was a survivor of extended trauma. At the end of the war, he was liberated and found his way to America.

As I grew up and developed a world perspective from my life experience, I came to understand that the secrecy represented the archetypical pattern of our family. This archetype was in place to pay homage to what came before. This homage possibly represented the sacrifice and the unthinkable things my father had to see and experience. As I have had time to reflect, I also believe this secrecy is a composite of many other factors.

So, even though the dinner happened more than thirty years after the war, I have come to see that the war was very much present in every aspect of what happened at the table. It not only governed the pattern of my interaction with my father, it also was operative on my parents' relationship and how it had evolved over the preceding years. The endurance and survival had made central to my parents the social and cultural imperatives of the forties, fifties, sixties, and seventies—with the implicit goal of striving for a better life for themselves and their children. In order for that to happen, they had to leave the past behind and look forward. The past, remaining unresolved and as inaccessible as it was, continued to be reenacted in countless ways.

This secrecy also seemed to define the parameters and, because unexamined at the time, to create limits for my future. The choices I would make—and the expectations I believed myself required to meet—were defined in these terms for many years. They were ultimately diminished by my overwhelming and unquenchable curiosity to find my own sense of identity, normalcy, and life balance.

In the chapters that follow, I chart that path, especially in terms of the progression of my ability to care for patients as I have grown and cleared the negative effects of these early childhood events.

The next chapter in particular expands upon my early confusion and emotional turmoil. Thereafter, I do not chart my path in strict chronological order; it is in an order that identifies thematic benchmarks in my personal and professional growth.

My path has taken me to research that illuminates my own experience and heightens my sensitivity and empathy for those I serve. I have been fortunate to find the right personal resources at the right time—as well as information and ideas that have brought profound relevant insight to me. I have seen in particular that the whole human business of self-regulation, of finding the appropriate response to life's web of experience, can be illuminated by ferreting out and understanding some fascinating science, which I explore as we go.

What's at least as important, though, is that this process has ultimately made me progressively more empathic with my patients, who bring their life stories with them when they come to me for treatment. How that came to be follows. If my story serves to make my readers, including my patients, become more curious, more empowered to make good decisions, and less self-judging as they look at their own lives and experiences, I will have more than met my goal in telling it.

3

My Father, the Steward

Not long after the Saturday night dinner described in the preceding chapter, I experienced another side of my confusion, frustration, and tension. My father was the central character, but this time it also involved my friends.

I grew up in a typical New Jersey suburb in the 1970s. On our street, my sister and I hung out with a lot of kids our ages. This was my community. This was home more than the school I attended was. It was home more than my house was. I could ride my bike, go into the woods around our home with other neighbors, build tree house forts, and create dams in the local streams with rocks and fallen branches. It was a great place to grow up.

The life I had led up to that point was far from the Vietnam War, civil unrest, recession, inflation, and other things that the adults of the late 1960s and early 1970s had to deal with. Little League baseball and other periodic afterschool activities were not as prevalent as they are today, so this neighborhood was a big part of what shaped and gave positive energy to my life.

I needed the neighborhood as my source of safety and freedom and connection with friends. Though Vietnam was far away, I was frequently confused, frustrated, and tense inside our house. There, between fairly long intervals of peace, my parents fought. Listening to the argument and its deep verbal cuts made me wince. Yet, no matter the duration or the intensity of the argument, they always got back together, seeming to resume life where it had left off. I was left, frightened, trying to make what sense I could of it. Although their fights seemingly had nothing to do with me, they were never referred to afterward. I was left to try to make sense of what happened.

I felt an instinctive impulse to hover like a silent referee. My coping strategy was to anticipate a plan if the action got out of control. I also felt the responsibility to console my mother. The verbal barrages often followed the complaints I often heard her expressing to my father. "You're never home." "Where have you been?" My father's workaholic sales schedule often kept him away from home for extended times or present for a small part of the day when he was working locally. His absence was the source of many of my parents' arguments. Though I imagined supplying my mother's needs in his absence, my combination of curiosity and fear did nothing to inform how I might do that. Instead, unable to control, console, or anticipate, the only thing I could count on was escaping outside with my friends.

My friends would come over to visit; we had a basketball court on the driveway and a front yard with trees planted in such a way that space was allowed for a perfectly shaped baseball diamond. Although the trees sometimes got in the way, our yard had more open space than our neighbor's yards did. It became the natural hub where we would play baseball, football, or soccer.

Sometimes it seemed that my friends came over with a greater interest in having a conversation with my father than playing sports. As a salesman, my father was most adept at conversation. In the presence of my friends, he showed none of the behavior that so often characterized his interactions with my mother. What I saw was someone taking on the role of sage or steward of life. He would hold forth on how my friends might maximize their life potential right from the present moment. He would ask them their interests and how they thought those interests would fit into the big picture of life. My friends seemed intoxicated by his vision for them, and welcomed the idea that an adult saw something in them that was larger than they could picture for themselves. As he shared his lore and vision, he spoke in flowery language and punctuated his words with sweeping gestures. At times, I also wondered whether my friends were just there to be entertained rather than to receive his validation and counsel.

What I remember feeling about these gatherings was self-consciousness, an automatic need to hover. Instead of just being fifteen, focused in the moment, and going with the flow of such gatherings, I would simply become a cautious and silent spectator, as if on duty for anything embarrassing or uncomfortable. Inwardly, I felt I was the guardian of the process, paying close attention and keeping everyone in line and convivial, even though I didn't at all feel empowered to manage any uncomfortable moments.

I remember one such conversation a group of my friends had with my father on our driveway. The topic was our individual and collective futures and the career path that each of us was destined for. At fifteen and only in my first year of high school, my vision of a career path was cloudy at best. However, one of my closest friends was one of the most driven students I knew. Tom's father was a mechanical engineer and had a great stable job with Bell Labs. Tom seemed to have his life all planned out to follow in his father's footsteps.

Tom was sharing his story with my father as if he were making a case for the affirmative on the school debate team. As he methodically described the details of his planned future, I listened in earnest and found myself going along with Tom's argument. I found his position convincing, but I really just wanted the conversation to end because we had planned to ride our bikes to a friend's house a couple of streets over. We were late for a swimming date, and I could see my father warming to this juicy opportunity to hold forth.

Tom was into his story. I could tell by the way he spoke that he felt confident and assured of his future. It was clear as day that his motives were more than just taking an easy ride following in his family's career path. I was actually jealous because he had such clarity and unbounded confidence about the next stages of his life.

We all listened without saying a word. As Tom was finishing up his argument, I was hoping I could put an end to this conversation so we could go swimming. Instead, my father launched into a point-by-point commentary on why Tom's logic was terribly flawed. He said, "Well, you know, what you are going to learn will be obsolete by the time you graduate! All the time and effort you will be putting into your degree, all the money that you are going to invest in your education will be simply wasted."

I should have been used to my father's style, the unilateral self-assurance, but I was mortified not because of what my father said but because of his seeming complete lack of sensitivity and compassion for Tom's ideas. He didn't stop there.

He said, "Tom, with all of your people skills and intelligence, you will do much better studying to be a lawyer. You will be able to call your own shots, and your life as an engineer won't even come close to matching the opportunities the legal profession will give you." As if finishing an oral argument, he exclaimed, "You need to consider this! You will thank me in twenty years!"

The look on Tom's face was one of puzzlement. On one hand, he looked dumbfounded with his mouth slightly open, but he also had a little smile. I didn't know if this was because he was actually considering what my father was suggesting or if he was just chuckling to himself. I felt really awkward; I also felt responsible for keeping the conversation under control, not going off track with my father's energy. I just had to break the pregnant pause, and tried coming to Tom's rescue.

I said, "Well, his father and uncle also have a side engineering business, and Tom will have more than enough opportunity."

My father did not even bother to respond to my point. I felt completely ignored, thrown under the bus. He simply resumed pursuit of his closing clincher, this time looking up close at me. "We, as a country, are shipping everything overseas. Unless Tom wants to move to a third world country to work in an overseas factory, he will do what I am saying. I know I am right."

I didn't mind if this sage wisdom would ultimately direct Tom to a more fulfilling life path. I even told myself I didn't mind being thrown under the bus. I was used to my father's dismissal of my opinions. From prior experience, I had learned not to challenge his comments or defend mine since he seemed to relish making me see the error in my logic. I just wanted the haziness in my head and sour sick feeling in my body to go away. Despite my vigilance, I was powerless to make this happen.

Just as with my experience at the dinner table, I was searching for resolution and some release from the tension and mental paralysis. I couldn't open my mouth. I was secretly furious. I wanted to scream, "These are my friends and my community! I put up with the disharmony in the house. Do I have to put up with it out here too? Out here, we play and have fun. Your rules don't apply! This is my territory! Out here, we make the rules. You are taking away my lifeline!"

Instead, these words were merely rehearsed in my head. I made my private adaptation and peace in the moment, as I always did in such situations, as my father finally turned and walked up the driveway to the house. Breathing a sigh of relief, I hopped on my bike and set out with my friends for the swim that had been deferred by this drama.

As I have reflected on this event and others like it, I have made peace with the thoughts and feelings that were so inescapable at the time. I can look back and gain clarity and understanding by seeing what fueled my emotions and the beliefs behind those misguided rules I made with myself that certainly had not been discussed and agreed upon with my parents or my friends. It was kind of a pact I had made with myself to negotiate the hard feelings I had come in contact with over time. The hurt I was experiencing was too painful to do anything about—other than to deny and adapt.

Over time, my thoughts about my father have changed. For one, he did have a good hunch about the future of the economy. What my father was saying about outsourcing was actually prophetic and ahead of its time, considering it was 1976. It's amazing that he had seemed to intuit the shape of things to come with the state of manufacturing in America and to have been confident that if Tom had become an engineer his job might well have ended up being outsourced. Perhaps it was pure luck.

His apparent brilliance in seeing things so clearly did nothing to connect him with me. It did nothing to meet my need to feel valued, to feel confident in my own thinking and decisions, or to be understood in my longing to escape the mental and emotional prison to whose confines I had so painfully adapted. It had exactly the opposite effect. Instead I was trapped in a subjective state that painted a world without any exit strategy.

I noted in my Saturday night dinner story that my subsequent path led me to becoming informed about my father's life. I noted that his life in Europe during World War II was off limits for my parents in a big way. When the story that they did choose to share was getting to something significant, they couldn't go on any further.

It was as if the memories and their implications were too much to bear.

This perspective has allowed me to observe and recast how my parents, especially my father, dealt so incompletely with the feelings about his emotionally charged childhood. I have come to see that the frozen state I often found myself in was simply a different version of the frozen state of secrecy and denial that drove my father's behavior in its own way. He did not intend to hurt me. Given the circumstances, he simply couldn't do any better. His discussion with Tom actually drove that point home. Though the dynamics were different, his behavior and his attitude toward Tom were just as authoritarian and dysfunctional as they were in dealing with me.

My father's past was never resolved, and no resolution was attempted. I feel I can say this without knowing his complete history. I have learned that the frustration he had with me was not really much about me. Yes, it is tempting to imagine what might have occurred if my family had felt comfortable openly sharing the war stories and details of my father's survival. I can only guess the impact that understanding would have had on the rest of my life. That was not to be, but I have still found a path to compassion and empathy.

The process of finding this path has shaped my personal life and my professional career. The path continues to have scientific, psychological, emotional, and spiritual dimensions—for me and those I serve.

As we move into the next chapters and a description of my professional education and early career, you will see my initial lack of strategies to cope, see the different parts of me working together as well as at cross purposes, as I gradually came to look at my work as more than technique, customer service, or even "effective communication." In many ways, this progression parallels my personal progression toward self-knowledge.

I came to see and respect that the range of needs and expectations of my patients was wide—and that there was no one-size-fits-all approach. It was not all about me and my heroic vigilance or responsiveness. Some patients want to get to the point, get it over with, and just do it already. Some under-share what is happening with them; some overshare and dramatize. Neither of these two self-regulating strategies is right or wrong. The answer is different for every patient, even though the answer may be hidden. In any case, my role has become one of opening the windows of insight, based on my personal experience, observation, and study—and knowing that the answer is not ultimately up to me.

In these first three chapters, I have taken what has sometimes felt like a big risk. I trust the content of my stories explains why. It did not always feel safe for me as a boy to share and lay claim to the value of my experience and thoughts. Yet it has seemed increasingly necessary to reclaim this voice, my vulnerability and uncertainty notwithstanding, if I wanted to be who I really am. In a way my choice to share is nothing greater than what I expect and value most from patients who want to reclaim their own power, transcend their anxieties, take a seat in the dental chair regardless, and put their trust in the personal as well as professional transaction that is about to occur.

Having put these stories into what seemed to be the most significant context, I leave off further analysis and trust the reader to make obvious inferences about their impact and influence on the personal and professional trajectory of my life, my thoughts, my emotions, my choices, my impulses, and my still-emerging perspective.

4

FINDING MY WAY IN DENTISTRY

In college, I worked part-time in a dental office and a dental lab. I was leaning toward a career in dentistry and wanted to see if the profession was going to be right for me.

My main experience was working for several summers in a nearby group practice office as a chair-side assistant. My training there was orchestrated by several coworkers—all female. Male assistants were uncommon at the time. They were seasoned veterans who had been working in what were the golden years of the profession. Each of them had at least thirty years of experience, starting in the 1950s.

They were professionals, and they eagerly wanted to show me exactly how things were done. The instruments were to be arranged in a precise way in a precise location. They were to be held and transferred to the dentist in a very specific way. What they wanted me most to know was that there was a very special bearing I needed to assume. As chair-side assistant, I needed to make myself as nearly invisible as possible—and certainly not be heard. This was a first principle of competency. All verbal and nonverbal communication (gestures, posture, and facial expression) needed to have the tone of a Tibetan bell. I was to act like the ball boy or ball girl who picks up tennis balls during professional play: retrieve them and return to your place smartly. It would be the ideal if I could be invisible—even when I was just a few inches from the patient.

This unquestioned principle carried over to my approach to applying to dental school at Fairleigh Dickinson University, where I was an undergraduate. I wanted to strike the presumed right tone in order to have the best chance of admission, which was quite competitive. I went about the process in a very intentional and deliberate way.

Dr. Goldman (as with other persons described in this book, not her real name), a dentist at the group practice where I worked, was a recent graduate of FDU. Further, she knew the graduate admissions director there. She agreed to review my application essay. I presented a piece that I thought would strike the perfect tone: a compelling and engaging narrative that extolled my accomplishments in high school and college and explained why my background and goals in the profession made me more than worthy of acceptance.

Dr. Goldman read my essay and said everything was fine, except for one big glaring problem. In the essay, I had referred to my experience as a dental assistant. I had explained that I wanted to emulate the dentists I worked with to provide "care that was not painful." Ouch!

"Painful," she said, looking me in the eye, "is a red-flag word. In dentistry, professionals do not talk about the care we provide as causing pain. If you are going to be a professional, you need to start thinking and acting like one. You need to deflect, and minimize this, because it's just not done. I know for sure that the admissions office will not be impressed."

I made the necessary change of wording in the application. I believe my edited text referred to "making patients comfortable" and "creating confidence in successful treatment," or something equally bland. Despite it all, I still found it a shock how the mental attitude and behavioral mode I had previously assumed on the job was going to be completely necessary on the job and off. The mere mention of pain was to be forever off-limits.

I had worked hard to get to that point in my life, and I wasn't about to put my education and future career in jeopardy. I rationalized that if acquiring the professional title of DMD was going to prevent me from openly talking about pain, then so be it. I would accept the tradeoff. I decided to go along with the program; it was too great a risk to bring my questions up among fellow students or professional colleagues. I never asked for—and thus never received—a satisfactory explanation.

I plunged into the dental curriculum with a single mission: a mastery of the requisite science and a grasp of the technology and development of the necessary skill. I absorbed—or at least went along with—the whole prevailing ethos regarding the attitude I needed to take and the way I should be present with patients.

When I began my professional career, I found that playing this role allowed me entrance into the club. I simply modeled what I did after the received standard model—what I had seen and heard. I did what I had seen done in dental school. It served me well in several of my first real jobs as a licensed dentist, including the group practice where I was an assistant for several years before striking out on my own.

Even when I struck out on my own, it continued to serve me well. My new practice grew, and I received broad positive feedback about my services. Patients came and remained with me. I was aware of the conscious choice I had made and tried to resign myself to the fact that being in the club and acting within this preassigned role was part of what goes with the territory of being a dentist.

The paradigm was reinforced in many ways. For example, there were the professional magazines and publications. Most of the newsmagazines featured (and still do!) articles that addressed marketing, patient relations, record keeping, the office environment, ten "dos and don'ts" for this or that. Or they reported exciting new technology in equipment or peripheral electronics that would make actual work less uncomfortable, more permanent, more efficient, more aesthetically pleasing, and more cost-effective. The conferences and workshops advertised in these publications were chiefly about such specifics as personnel management, acquiring new patients, using new technology, or owning versus renting your office space. And much of the space in these publications was devoted to advertising everything from equipment to toothpaste. It was all about the business and building your practice.

I can't say the information contained in these publications—or the study and professional practices I adopted—were irrelevant or useless. I often found good ideas for the tactical and logistic details of my practice. And I still do. Here's an example of my experience with one particular practice dimension that I pursued for an extended period in the 1990s—and the ultimate outcome.

One area of practical concern for me was how the physical aspects of the office itself—the arrangement of space, the location of various functions, the flow of traffic, the colors and other design elements—could collectively influence the psychological state of a patient walking in the door. I wanted my dental space to be efficient and "user-friendly."

You may be familiar with the sliding door that separates the patients in the waiting room from the rest of the dental office. This door, sometimes barely more than a peephole in some offices, can certainly be justified on the grounds that it manages the flow that is required for patients in various stages of their visit. Managing this flow and maintaining privacy are important for any dental office regardless of their practice philosophy; there needs to be latitude for personal taste and preferences in the details.

At that time, I had quite a large sliding door in my office. I felt it often served only to further distance the patient and the dental team. Yes, it may have made the situation safer for some, but I wondered if it could also send the message: *We are in control here. We decide whether the door is open or not. What goes on behind the door is strictly ours to determine. You enter by permission of management only. We are we, and you are you.* This did not seem like a good business message.

At about that time, such considerations as the sliding door issue were leading to a rapid expansion of the specialty field of interior professional design, especially office design. Much more conscious attention was being given to traffic patterns, location of work centers, and creating a match between function and the feel of every corner of the office. And the applied science of ergonomics, the design of equipment for the workplace, was expanding rapidly. The goal of ergonomics was to maximize productivity by reducing human fatigue and discomfort, and my office was ripe for assessment.

With respect to the sliding door issue, current ergonomic thinking was coming to favor breaking down physical barriers in office space by using a more open floor plan. Yet, with respect to dental offices, the majority of new office design projects directed the movement of flow based upon the existence of a front desk with an open floor plan in the outer space.

In the late 1990s, Dr. William Dickerson wrote *Front Desklessness.* Written by a practicing dentist, the book challenged the central front desk theme. Its main premise was that patients should come first; a front-desk-centered office cannot manage the flow of patient traffic in the best fashion. Dr. Dickerson's way to put the patient first was radical: throw out the whole front desk—not just the wall that held the peephole. Instead, move all logistics from the front to the back where the patient care was provided. This model would not just enable better patient care, it would take advantage of rapidly emerging information technology. Computers were making it possible to have all the necessary information fully networked and immediately available in every workspace.

Although the design of the physical facility was a central subject of *Front Desklessness*, Dr. Dickerson also proposed that the real key to the success of the design involved changing staff roles and responsibilities so as to best adapt to it. For example, he suggested changing the usual role of chair-side assistants. These persons would now be called patient care coordinators.

The staff would be chosen and trained or retrained to provide both chair-side and front-desk-like functions. The position was more of a concierge who would coordinate the patient's visit from start to finish. Instead of the traditional process where the tasks are generally delegated to several different staff members, the patient care coordinators would handle everything, including patient questions and follow-up.

This concept really appealed to me, but I never did make the necessary changes required by the model. It just seemed too daunting in terms of time and money and staff retraining to make the transition. Something that had yet to be fully tested elsewhere— and would require turning my practice on its head—was a step too far for me. And it appeared that my staff members were not prepared psychologically for such a radical shift. I became much more conscious of the importance of details when it came to designing a patient-friendly office environment, but I chose to play it safe and conform to what was known to work, however imperfectly.

My inquiry into best practices with Dr. Dickerson also led me to search out other experts. I read their books, went to their courses, and even hired one group to personally guide me for a year using their data-management and goal-setting system. What all these resources had in common was an insistence on the importance of focusing on customer service. Dentistry was a business, and best business practices were to be applied here just as in any other business. I should therefore think in marketing terms: value and quality of customer service was the benchmark.

These experiences were never without usefulness. Implementing certain strategies no doubt helped my practice grow, and the way I was working seemed to more than suffice for a sizeable segment of my patients who regularly thanked me and expressed appreciation. I still use some of the business systems and practice logistic efficiencies I learned through my studies and consultations, and they serve me well.

As the preceding pieces of my life make clear, this addressed only part of my character and temperament. I call that part the reluctant conformist. Another part of me was telling me there was something missing. If my life work was going to work for me, this part told me it had to involve a more authentic and less production-oriented model of professional interaction: dentist with staff, dentist with patients, staff with patients. It made me question the organizational and leadership principles I was trying to follow. To this part of me, these principles seemed to have been cut and pasted from a generic corporate human resources playbook. They were actually antithetical to being a true professional on my own terms. This part told me I was just repeating a version of practice that tended toward a paternalistic hierarchy with an implicit condescension toward patients that I had learned unconsciously in dental school and seen at work in the practice where I originally assisted. It wanted to tell me that such a model might be fine for others—but not for me.

On the other hand, my other part saw that the relationship model would be one that would make dental care feel far less threatening and safer to obviously anxious or phobic patients, and also those whose relaxed appearance belied a more complex state of mind when they came into the office. Through my life experiences, such as those described in the first three chapters, I related to these patients. It was that simple. This part of me intuited that, beneath appearances, a lot was going on for a large segment of my patients. And it was a much bigger deal than most of what I was actually doing took into account. It was where the action was for this part of me.

The following chapter describes how this inner dialogue continued as I worked to create the ideal environment by trying different variations on how I might support the patient's experience with emerging technology and complementary adjuncts to conventional care.

5

THE HUMAN FACTOR

While following the prevailing business paradigm of the time in order to develop a "best practices" business model, to practice effectively, and to keep up with the latest technology, a part of me never stopped struggling with the way I had been strictly trained to consider patient behavior. This training had begun during the dental school application process; it ran uninterrupted through dental school and to providing treatment in the office where I worked prior to setting out on my own twenty years ago. So it was only natural that this part of me followed to my own practice, even down to how I should design the physical layout of the office to create a flow of activity that would partition the patient's experience from watching the technical details or examining the implements being used. The goal was to manage the patient's experience to minimize the risk of negative reactions.

While I was under the scrutiny of my dental educators and subsequent employers, I found myself observing standard protocol since I was not in my own territory. On one hand, this checklist training made sense because trying to take into account and respond to the wide array of patient behaviors seemed to be unfeasible at best and unproductively risky at worst. I was qualified as a technician, not a psychologist. Just deal with the task at hand. Once on my own, I could make choices for myself, but not while I was in someone else's employ.

The problem with being a "mechanic" was that, for a large part of me, this was far more than car repair. The car—in this case, the patient—was not a set of mechanical parts that didn't have any thoughts or feelings and couldn't express itself. I was dealing with a living organism. So the patient was both a "car" and a human being at the same time. I felt hard put to do double-duty. Some patients' successful care most definitely required me to balance the technical and customer service end and be sensitive to the anxieties and concerns that many patients brought with them. I needed to treat the tooth—and the needs, wants, and desires of the individual attached to the tooth. My sensitivity made it a real challenge to do so as if these were two distinct and separable activities.

My patients brought their days in with them. We all live in a stressful, anxious culture, and I have spent my entire professional career practicing in central New Jersey, a part of this country that seems to run on stress to an exceptional degree. This is a busy place that requires people to be constantly aware of time management. You can certainly see this by the way the population drives on local roads and highways. People seem to be always late. Nearly everyone seems impelled to drive fast—pushing well past posted speed limits on nearby Interstate 78, taking risks with passing on two-lane county roads with no distance to spare—while furtively checking cell phones for messages (use of cell phones while driving is illegal in New Jersey). Customers, whether at the bank, buying tires for their cars, or dealing with anyone on the other side of the counter, can be very curt and impatient. So can those on the other side of the counter. To have a life and fit everything in for some, things have to be done yesterday. I guess that's why there are so many fast food restaurants here.

I noticed this cultural ethos manifesting itself in my office from the very start. At least once a day, while I was in the process of beginning an appointment, making a consciously relaxed and measured entry into the room, or offering as casual a transition as possible into the present moment for the patient, some patients seemed on the way to the next business appointment or texting on their iPhone while offering the briefest acknowledgments of my presence. Some would quickly ask about a tooth or comment on some irrelevant subject or situation. A lot of the time, the impatient or insistent behavior challenged the resources of my staff members who handle the administration functions.

My receptionist would report situations at least weekly where someone had called for an immediate appointment to materialize out of thin air. I appreciated that many patients might have a legitimate emergency or need to squeeze the rest of their day's needs in order to honor the appointment, but it often seemed as if we were faced with the challenge of trying to accomplish several days' worth of dentistry in a few hours.

Of course, not all patients created drama for themselves and my team—and certainly not to the same degree. Most have set aside the rest of their life and are ready to put their attention to the here and now. I have no actual basis for firsthand comparison with how things might be for dentists elsewhere in this country. Perhaps my colleagues in other places would report the same thing I do.

The anxious behavior I observed did not seem occasioned by the prospect of imminent dentistry, as opposed to the prospect of a relaxing massage. Its presence was more like an additional generalized challenge regardless of whether the patient had any basic anxiety about dentistry. It is more like ambient noise without any conscious awareness. And whether patients were presenting themselves as nervous or casual, the larger social environmental context had its influence. Its influence affects how readily patients can become numb when anesthesia is applied and the ability to relax during treatment.

My patients could be divided into two camps when it comes to beginning treatment. Though they were offering two distinct types of observable behavior, they manifested the same underlying emotional states.

First, there were those who made no attempt to hide that they were focused on readying themselves for what was about to happen. Whether by exaggeratedly fidgeting for the right body position in the chair, repeatedly fine-tuning the position of the head and mouth before I was ready to look inside, or offering only head movement replies to my questions, it was clear they had a one-point unspoken program with no room for distractions: "Okay, doc. Just do what you gotta do!"

Some patients presented themselves in quite the opposite way. Rather than showing impatience or anxiety, they seemed "too cool for school." They were ready for chitchat, going on to the point where I found myself needing to redirect their attention to the business at hand. For these patients, though, I had a more subtle challenge. The opening gambits, where they engaged readily in small talk and seemed open, ready, and available, would give way to a stoic stiffening up, even more so than what my first category of patients would show. They often turned completely mum and uncommunicative well before I had inserted anything or even taken a look in their mouth, which would otherwise end the talking. They went to the other end of the communication spectrum. If I asked generic questions to help me stay connected and to guide my process (How is this for you? Are we good to keep going?), I couldn't be sure of their responses.

Much of what I did at this time was a seat-of-the-pants assessment of how best to continue. I was playing the role of an amateur dental detective. Incommunicative patients were like star witnesses to the situation, but they wouldn't testify. I needed their testimony—or I had to go on what I could physically observe or an X-ray could tell me. X-rays or physical examinations helped, but I also needed cooperative witnesses. Absence of cooperation—whether deliberate or whether the patient simply could not recall or describe something—worked against the best interests of both of us. It's an ironic coincidence that there is a technical term called "arresting" the decay, which is meant to describe how we would stabilize the tooth while cleaning out the decay. Without the witness, making the "arrest" is much more problematic. Often patients seemed to freeze.

Of course, what I have described as two distinct reactions to an impending unknown might better be seen as occurring on a spectrum and also with varying degrees of prominence. Some patients present some combination of both. Though one of these two reactions seems to be part of nearly every patient's behavior, many patients have only very little of it. They might not relate to this discussion at all, but my clinical experience is that many patients fall clearly into one of these two broad categories or present some combination of both behaviors. They all show some mental and emotional vulnerability, a heightened and unique sensitivity to dentistry, a sensitivity that may be suppressed or sedated or consoled, but not removed.

Given that just about everyone carries the stress and ambient anxiety of the culture, whether in New Jersey or anywhere else, I early on wanted to see what might be more valuable to me: the factors that determine individual behavior and account for individual differences in behavior, thought patterns, and feelings that my range of patients brought. Common sense would tell me that a patient in overall excellent health arriving for routine cleaning and examination would not come in with the same mental and emotional state as someone with extreme pain, chronic debilitating condition, or a recent family tragedy. One would be more relaxed, the other tense.

I did not see such a simple correlation between the current life circumstance of a patient and his or her behavior in my office. It seemed to make no difference whether a patient was healthy or whether the planned treatment was going to be simple, brief, and painless, or complex, lengthy, and discomforting. And it seemed to make no difference whether this was a first-time visit or an appointment with a longtime patient. It also seemed to make no difference whether they reported having a good or bad day. Some patients were anxious, hyper, and outgoing; others were relaxed, stoic, or withdrawn. Some did quick about-faces in their behavior in the middle of treatment; others had a constant demeanor throughout.

They all had the same basic anatomy and physiology when it came to the area involved in dentistry. The environment of the office and operatory was always essentially the same. I was wearing a white coat for one and all, and I made it a point to present myself in the same predictable manner. What were the variables? How did essentially the same set of stimuli generate such a range of responses? Perhaps if I could identify and understand the variables, I could isolate the key.

I wondered if a possible explanation might be found in the unique sensitivity of each patient's dental territory. Could they be subtly working to amplify or soften anxiety in ways that were not related to immediate environment or life circumstances? After all, where the work takes place is also a place where the many highly sensitive cranial nerves are readily activated. If I could understand how these nerves worked either separately or in concert, and then control the variables, I might be able to apply this understanding to my niche in operatory. I could enhance safety, connection, and trust in a way that was more limited by conventional approaches. This was to be the start of something big, the hunt for "tooth sense."

While the hunt was just beginning, I tried, hit-or-miss, a wide range of personal approaches and technological tactics. I invested in the quietest drill. I tweaked the details of managing the patient's anticipation of the shot, carefully controlling water flow in the back of the throat, even adjusting the chair position perfectly. I spent more time and went into more detail in describing what I was doing as I went, checking frequently to make sure the patient was comfortable.

I also began to incorporate various support devices, ancillary products, and other services to aid in this approach. Whether it was the administration of nitrous oxide as a mild sedative to "take the edge off," a warm moist towel before care, special pillows, or even a fully integrated TV multimedia system called the Dental Couch Potato, whereby the patient could watch a TV program or movie to take his or her mind away from the goings-on, I was ready to try it.

I also incorporated more natural products like aromatherapy, color therapy glasses, and homeopathic remedies. I tried dental lasers and an electronic relaxation device called a Biomodulator. Yet knowing that I had gone far beyond what was even available through most dental catalogs, and still experiencing a range of results from good to counterproductive, I wondered whether the more esoteric the device or product, the less successful the outcome. I eventually concluded that my quest for the silver bullet, so to speak, was following a false trail.

Getting the kind of responses, from what I had perhaps naively thought would be no-brainer helping tactics, left me confused to say the least. The deeper impact of this also had me take pause, and even had me fall back upon the simple task- and results-oriented service paradigm in which I had been trained.

Still, the longer my underlying frustration continued, the more motivated I was to find something more fundamentally grounded in science to illuminate my path. I found myself spending more and more of my spare time researching the anatomical territory where I worked—the structures and functions of the oral cavity. In short, how everything in this complex area really worked. Let me explain what I mean by "anatomical territory" and note the specific questions I began to ask.

The teeth, tongue, mouth, throat, and neck—and all the bones, muscles, and connective tissue that connect them and hold them in place—work in concert and communicate together through our nervous system to regulate the sensing and response of this critical region. It seemed to me that the total symphony of activity played in such a way as to exercise an outsized influence on more than just the health of our teeth. Wasn't there something about its location, its sensitivity, and the process of its component parts working together that had some function in regulating all mental and emotional tone—in effect, the quality of life and its relationships? It was as if the whole production involved a special sense that had neurological, psychological, and emotional components. It required a new name. Nothing I knew seemed to capture it; this territory seemed to carry an embedded network of signals that affected human expression in general. I chose to call it "tooth sense," which seemed imprecise. But what I was describing seemed not precise. So as I have come to better identify and describe what I am referring, I have kept the term, absent anything better.

At any rate, whatever I would call it, I wanted to see if identifying, describing, and exploring its workings wouldn't help make my menu of treatment tactics more grounded in science and therefore more applicable. From the outset, I felt that "tooth sense" was not a conscious process or activity. It was certainly nonverbal, and it didn't seem subject to conscious influence.

And it was not really one thing. It was an emotional and neurological activity that proceeded as a byproduct of a number of structural and functional oral cavity workings under certain conditions. By analogy, it resembled what I think of when I think of "mind." Mind is not a thing. "Mind" refers to how our consciousness experiences the activity of the brain and the rest of the nervous system—an activity, not a thing. Likewise, "tooth sense" refers more specifically to how we experience the workings of the oral cavity and surrounding area.

As such, one's tooth sense is shaped basically by physical sensations and the tone of our emotional responses to these sensations. It is the component of what is activated when a certain stimulus—a perceived threat or risk, for instance—is present. Because dentistry occurs in a vulnerable and sensitive area, and involves the patient giving up control and needing to trust an unknown, it plays a big part in shaping an appropriate evaluation of the situation in the moment (Is it safe or dangerous?), and thus on self-regulation, decision making, staying in the present moment, and being socially engaged with others. Tooth sense can be a powerful ally. Or it can lead to "missed cues" and outsized reactions to perceived threats when none are present.

This was how I came, however tentatively, to frame and describe "tooth sense." And this formulation has mostly turned out to be the way I still see it. What has evolved is insight into a more refined understanding of the how, why, and where of its workings. That, of course, is what the rest of the book explores.

It turned out I was going to be in luck in my early investigations. It was at this time, around 2000, that the results of quite a bit of scientific research in the fields of evolutionary biology and neurobiology were appearing, not just in the scientific journals, but also in popular literature. I was very interested. This work was not directly relating to dentistry, but it might, I thought, shed some light on the subtle dynamics I was observing every day. I had never seen these dynamics addressed in the dental scholarly journals. In fact, the research appealed to me precisely because it was not limited to dental matters. All the books that came my way seemed to be reaching for the bigger picture of human behavior and why humans act, think, and feel the way they do—and not just in the dental chair. They were each in their own way reaching to resolve part of the riddle of "human vulnerability," our susceptibility to mistaken reading of and response to experience, and misplaced fears, a susceptibility on the wiring and electrical activity of human anatomy and physiology, especially in the geographical area of my work, the oral cavity.

In my quest, I dug into a number of books and articles that were definitely not part of my dental school curriculum. Among those that spoke to me were: *Emotional Intelligence* by Daniel Goleman, PhD; *The Great Leap Forward* by Terence Davidson, PhD; *Healing Trauma: Attachment, Mind, Body, and Brain* by Daniel Siegel, MD, and Marion Solomon; and *Social Engagement and Attachment* by Stephen Porges, PhD. As you can see, none of these titles were about management of dental practices or pitches for the newest technology. The works of these authors represented in this list, and numerous others, became part of my growing bookshelf. The ideas and information contained in such sources intrigued me in their originality and potential for guidance to a deeper understanding of the dynamics of dentistry, and how best to practice it.

In the next four chapters, I share my ideas, how they evolved, and how, when taken as a whole, they have opened up a richer, more holistic perspective—and created an ongoing conversation with myself about the implications of these ideas. As I may repeat frequently, though it has altered in major ways the way I view and conduct my practice, it is still very much a work in progress. I am hereby opening up this ongoing process to any readers inclined to participate in the conversation.

6

CONSIDERING THE SCIENCE

Though I was now mostly casting a wider net of inquiry into the workings of "tooth sense," one not confined to dental research or science, I also found myself reviewing some old notes from my dental school days. I came across some striking old illustrations of the way the nervous system works in various parts of the body. These illustrations are portrayals of maps of the brain based upon the work of the prominent early twentieth-century Canadian surgeon Wilder Penfield, MD. These illustrations present a cartoon character called the cortical homunculus ("little man"). There are two cortical homunculi, shown in figures 1 and 2.

As you can see, these figures represent a scale model of a human drawn or sculpted to reflect the relative space human body parts occupy on the somatosensory cortex (figure 1) and the motor cortex (figure 2). In both figures, for example, because human lips, mouth, head, and hands have relatively more sensory or motor neurons than other parts of the body, the homunculi illustrations have correspondingly large lips, mouth, head, and hands. Note that the motor homunculus looks quite similar to the sensory homunculus, but not exactly the same.

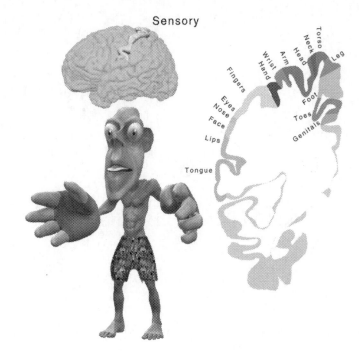

figure 1

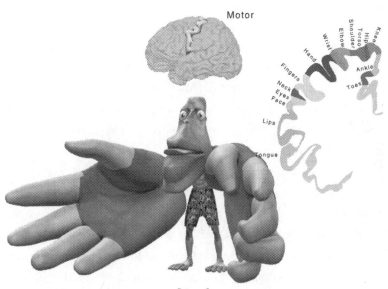

figure 2

Also, though not specifically shown in the illustrations, these sensitive areas of the oral cavity depict the response to touch. This system is quite complicated and as such is referred to as the somatosensory system. Although this system primarily depicts touch, it also is associated with the stimulus of temperature, proprioception (body position, movement), and pain. So it is no wonder that, in its workings, this overall somatosensory system creates a special set of challenging conditions for the practice of dentistry.

Reminded anew of this reality, I was also conscious that, as a hardwired situation, it applied to everyone. All humans with undamaged central nervous systems have the same basic anatomy and physiology. We are designed and wired for survival, so not every part of the body is set up to have the same sensitivity or reactivity. For example, the mouth is more critical to survival than the wrist; hence the mouth needs to assess touch, temperature, movement, and pain more sensitively than does the wrist. This has nothing to do with character or individual personality. It's a matter of automatic response to anything that presents itself as threatening. Yet the corollary to this situation is that the mouth and oral area is also more susceptible to outsize or inaccurate evaluation of what it senses.

But what none of this explained to me was this: Why did different patients have such different individual responses to what was essentially the same set of stimuli? Why didn't they exhibit similar physical responses to the same sensory experiences that I was presumably supplying in the environment of my office? What were the still unknown variables that I had not already sought to control—variables such as the office environment, the protocols, the techniques, and the way I presented myself or interacted—in short, all that I have described in the two previous chapters. What would account for the individual differences?

To better see what physiological mediators might be responsible for the differences in individual response, one of my investigations led to examining an action every patient performed many times during treatment. I became fascinated by how we swallow. Most of us take this simple process for granted—and it occurs between two thousand and three thousand times per day.

Swallowing is an especially significant activity when we are infants, when feeding is essentially the most important action we take to ingest nutrients and develop in every way. For this activity, we are deeply reliant upon those who care for us, especially our mothers. The quality of bond an infant and mother share exerts a strong influence on physical and emotional development. The training is handled via a nerve in the back of the mouth called the vagus nerve.

One of twelve cranial nerves, the vagus nerve starts in the brain and snakes its way down to service all the organs from the throat to the gut. The neural training that this nerve undergoes during the crucial early days, weeks, and months of life creates the vagal tone, a tone unique to each of us. This activity is associated with the parasympathetic nervous system, a part of our nervous system that works peripherally along with the sympathetic nervous system. The parasympathetic nervous system, as commonly understood, is inhibitory; it provides a "rest-and-withdrawal" complement to the "fight-or-flight" impulse supplied by the sympathetic nervous system when there is a perceived threat. A more detailed discussion of these components of the nervous system will come later in chapter 8, but this suffices at this point.

The degree of activity that the vagus nerve has within the parasympathetic nervous system is referred to as vagal tone—the unconscious emotional quality of how we experience changes of bodily functions such as the heart rate and other key functions. It regulates our speed and ability to override danger signals that turn out to be false alarms.

Coincidentally, I came across some interesting information about infant feeding, specifically the possible differences in early neurological and psychological development between bottle-fed and breast-fed infants. Taking place as it does in the anatomical neighborhood of the vagus nerve, this process might be experienced and recorded in memory in different ways for different infants. These differences might create different predispositions to reacting to safety or danger. I was excited to find out that whether an individual is breast-fed or formula-fed makes a significant difference in the quality of the vagal tone of an individual's emotional response.

Breast-feeding is a natural practice as old as motherhood itself. Many benefits derive from breast-feeding, including the swallow pattern. The breast-feeding swallow has been linked to the creation of a host of benefits that range from decreased bedwetting, decreased ear infections, and reduced future risk of sleep apnea. Still, quite early in the twentieth century bottle-feeding became—and largely remains—the favored method of feeding.

Though this preference is perhaps largely because bottle-feeding is simpler and more convenient from the parents' perspective, some research sought to support its benefits to infants as well. One study found that weaned babies slept a median of nine to ten hours at a stretch at every age after four months, and nursing babies slept in bouts of four to seven hours to the end of the second year. Weaning would thus be thought to be beneficial by reducing stress for the mother, allowing both mother and infant more regular and uninterrupted sleep.

Many, however, disagreed with this evaluation. Lactation consultant and researcher Marsha Walker, RN, has argued that such benefits are not only questionable, but, even if valid, trivial compared with the benefits of breast-feeding. She has written and spoken widely about the relationship between bottle-feeding and poor vagal nerve tone. Poor vagal tone, her research has shown, adversely affects the infant's physiological, mental, and social development.

Brian Palmer, DDS, has studied and reported extensively on how the breast-feeding swallow creates a stripping action that develops the perioral muscles (the muscles around the mouth). The quality of this action would seem clearly to influence the vagus nerve since the vagus nerve services the muscles immediately adjacent to the opening at the end of the mouth and the muscles extending into the pharynx, which is the cavity behind the nose and mouth.

Palmer also notes that bottle-feeding creates a vortex effect to the swallow in which there is a greater volume of fluid moving into the mouth than with breast-feeding. Due to the suction that is created in contact with an artificial nipple, there can be an adverse effect on how the palate forms. It may create a bubble palate (an unnatural engorgement of the palate). Whether or not this happens, the bottle-feeding sucking action prevents the perioral muscles and, by extension, the vagus nerve function from developing properly. Additionally, the stripping action associated with the breast-feeding swallow raises the position of the larynx, whereas the different action associated with bottle-feeding does not. By raising the larynx, the stripping action of breast-feeding creates a better-shaped palate (one less constricted and high) and develops the muscles in back of the mouth.

These considerations eventually led me to considerable speculation. In the interest of unfolding the story in chronological order, I'm saving that subject for the next chapter, where I will be introducing the function of the epiglottis.

Instead, I'd like to conclude this chapter by noting one additional related area of reported research that I found at the time. I discovered it while looking at other aspects of early childhood development—beyond the strictly neurological aspects that might be explicitly involved in the creation of vagal tone. I was also interested in the psychological aspects of development that take place in the first stages of life. I wondered how a mother's relationship with the infant—what is technically referred to as her social engagement—might influence, support, or inhibit the development of healthy vagal tone.

John Bowlby, PhD, and Mary Ainsworth, PhD, had done landmark research on this topic during much of the second half of the last century. They focused on the essential role that the primary caregiver has in meeting the first and most critical need of the newborn: the need to experience a deep connection and safety, to experience the world as a safe and trustworthy place. When such a positive sense is experienced, a foundation is laid for healthy development of the growing child's ability to accurately assess perceived threat, regulate reactivity, and eventually lead a richer and more secure adult life.

Such a positive outcome, they showed, depends on creating what they termed a "secure attachment" bond, achieved through the appropriate responsiveness of the mother. The behavior of the mother develops a sense of security and models such behavior on an unconscious level for the infant. They were especially interested in the effect of various patterns of parenting on the quality of this bond. They noted that this stage of development takes place within a relatively short period of time, probably little more than a year at the most. A mother has a critical window to create a secure attachment bond. It is critical because, as implied above, the quality she provides has everything to do with how the growing child is able to be with one's self—and, by extension, how that person will be able to "be" in all social situations, how that person is able to modulate responses in reaction to new environments and people who they will invariably need to negotiate with. If this need is not met, it does not disappear; it remains stored in memory as unfinished business.

While I was left unable to see a clear relationship between the quality of an infant's development of secure attachment and the development of vagal tone, I did not dismiss the possibility of a connection. Fortunately, new information would lead the way to a promising hunch about such a connection.

7

FOLLOWING A HUNCH

In the last chapter, I discussed some inherent vulnerability that all of us as humans share as infants. I noted my hunch—that the quality of the swallow pattern that each of us employs in feeding during the first year of life—may play a significant role in how we in all of later life sense and respond more generally to experience.

I happened to have several patients whose teeth showed significant and abnormal signs of wear, the kind of wear caused by grinding. It was no surprise that these patients all seemed to describe their lives as stressful. I was curious about the connection—and why patients would take out their daily stress on their teeth through grinding. This habit, known technically as bruxism, can wear teeth down, cause chipping, and even break teeth. The amount of load that this habit exerts on the teeth can slowly kill teeth or cause other associated problems with the bite and the gums. Somehow the profession has always been at a loss to stop this destruction.

In the absence of pain and other symptoms, the management protocol for this condition is to create a plastic device that covers and protects the teeth from this aggressive habit, which normally occurs at night. These dental devices, called bruxism appliances, are a useful preventive, but I have always been concerned that they represented a Band-Aid approach. They did not address or treat the underlying cause.

The exact mechanism by which bruxism occurs is not fully known, but it has typically been attributed in the dental profession to "psychosomatic disorder." It implies that psychological factors are involved, but it goes no further. Psychology was for mental health professionals. It was not part of the dental school curriculum or viewed as a useful field for what is essentially a technical matter. The other attribution of grinding was "structural problems." With this diagnosis, the goal of the dentist was to mitigate the effects of faulty structure, such as the bite, but not investigate the underlying anatomical or physiological causes. The emphasis was on the direct management of the given situation. For either diagnosis, we were taught to be "tooth carpenters" with a specialty analogous to storm damage repair. The dentist's job was to patch or repair—not to look at underlying structural problems that might have made particular sections of the building so readily susceptible to repeat damage.

Further, I found somewhat to my surprise that part of the science community sees significant benefits from bruxism. For example, the Japanese researcher Sadao Sato, DDS, and his Austrian colleague Rudolf Slavicek, PhD, proposed that bruxism was actually an excellent way to relieve stress. They looked at biochemical processes activated by grinding—processes that seem to improve functioning in the emotional center of the brain (the limbic area) and autonomic nerve function. They also looked at an overall decrease in stress load by looking at hormone blood levels and how stress hormones affect the hypothalamus, which coordinates the activity of the whole autonomic nervous system. If the premise of Sato and Slavicek was to be accepted, perhaps the wearing away of teeth was preferable to a heart attack.

As a dentist, though, I was not satisfied with the proposition that teeth are disposable on behalf of stress relief. I kept wondering about the process by which teeth came to be the mediators for expression of stress and negative emotions. The teeth were presumably not the direct cause of the anger, but they expressed it. If teeth fulfilled this function, was it also possible—maybe even likely—that other parts of the anatomy, especially parts served by the same cranial nerve group, could do the same? I was drawn to look more closely at the geographic neighbors to the teeth—the tongue, throat, and other organs—wondering whether they didn't also serve as mediators of expressions of emotion. I knew these organs were not serviced by the same cranial nerves in the cranial group, so I could only speculate, but I was drawn to do so.

I might not have gotten far in my pursuit of this idea if I had not come across some very intriguing detail about the actual stages involved in the swallowing process. What transpired from the time food entered the mouth until it left the throat was more complicated than I had recalled studying in school.

Briefly, here's how the swallow takes place. There are four distinct phases, each with a responsibility.

1st phase Oral Stage

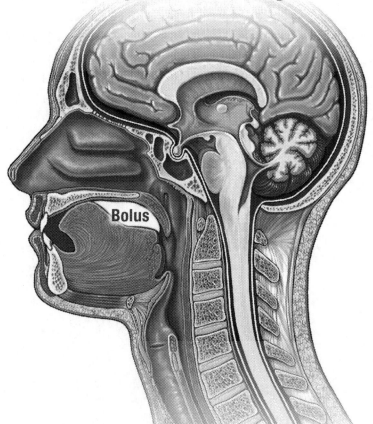

Bolus

The oral stage includes both the oral preparatory phase, and the oral transport phase.

2nd phase - Pharyngeal

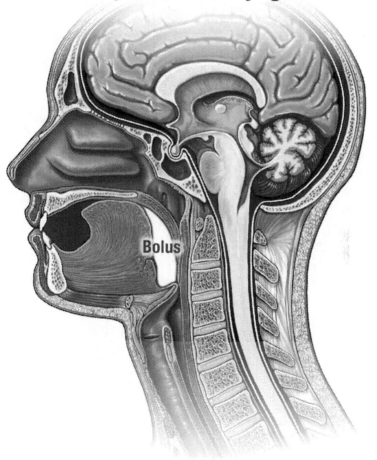

Bolus

3rd phase - Esophageal stage

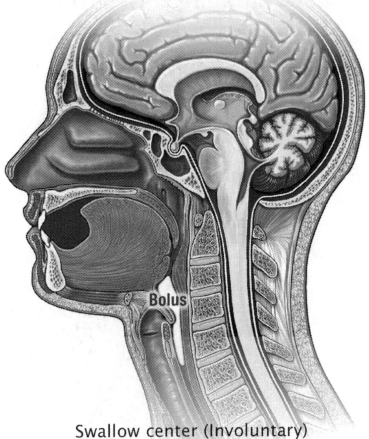

Bolus

Swallow center (Involuntary)

In this illustration, the first two stages are combined in the left figure. In the first, during the so-called oral preparatory phase, the food that is chewed, technically known as the bolus, is made small and round, and then properly positioned for transport. During the second or oral transport phase, the food bolus is transported from the the front (anterior) to the rear (posterior) part of the oral cavity. In the third or pharyngeal phase shown in the middle figure, the bolus starts its descent toward the rearmost part of the cavity known as the pharynx. The pharynx opens into the esophagus, which is the swallowing tube through which, in the fourth and final stage, the esophageal phase, illustrated in the right figure, the bolus is propelled to the stomach and the rest of the digestive system. The action in this fourth stage is automatic and unconscious propulsion through the reflexive movement known as peristalsis.

Of the four phases, the third or pharyngeal phase struck me as the most critical because of something that occurs there. The first two stages are performed consciously, or voluntarily. The fourth stage is unconscious, or involuntarily. The transition during the third stage in preparation for the fourth stage usually presents itself to the swallower as an all-or-nothing moment. You are about to give over conscious control of the process at this very moment. The nature of this transition should be familiar to anyone who has ever swallowed a pill or other substance that has not lent itself to being turned into a nice round and soft bolus. Is it ready to go down or not? Am I ready to execute? Do I spit it out or swallow it? How this seemingly all-or-nothing choice is made intrigued me.

What is especially significant is that this act of swallowing has been shown to happen between two thousand and three thousand times per day. That's at least twice per minute! If not executed properly, it can actually be life threatening. The Heimlich maneuver for dislodging trapped food or other matter is not widely taught without good reason. It is a well-known lifesaver. If we are not prepared or happen to be caught off-guard when this phase occurs, we risk choking and possible death if the bolus or liquid goes into the windpipe or trachea instead of the esophagus for further breakdown.

Also, what occurs in this pharyngeal phase is that other passageways into and out of the throat must be temporarily blocked as the pharynx becomes elevated in preparation of the bolus. The opening of a part of the pharynx called the oropharynx closes temporarily to keep all of the contents of the mouth from passing into the pharynx at once. Lastly, the openings to the auditory tubes, which lead into the ears, open during swallowing to relieve pressure.

As I looked at the various steps and stages of the swallow, specifically the all-or-nothing response of the pharyngeal phase, I wanted to see if I could identify the exact way this activity shifts from being conscious to involuntary. These two sets of stages are regulated by different nerve functions. The first two voluntary phases of the swallow are regulated by the central nervous system (CNS), essentially the brain and spinal cord. This master control system receives, integrates, stores, and retrieves sensory information in specific locations in the brain. The latter two involuntary phases are mostly regulated by the autonomic nervous system (ANS), the section of the nervous system that controls the involuntary actions of the muscles, heart, and glands. How does this shift occur? How does the vagal tone affect how this process is experienced? How might this tone affect the ability to deal with food, but also—by extension—the experience of dentistry? Finally, how does vagal tone affect how a person processes life itself?

I realized this was an exploration into seemingly esoteric territory, but I remained curious and kept looking. I researched a unique structure that prevents the contents of the mouth from going down the wrong way. A flap of cartilage (the epiglottis) covers the windpipe or trachea.

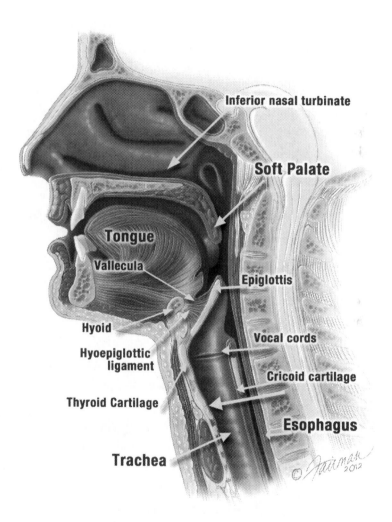

Inferior nasal turbinate

Soft Palate

Tongue

Vallecula

Epiglottis

Hyoid

Vocal cords

Hyoepiglottic
ligament

Cricoid cartilage

Thyroid Cartilage

Esophagus

Trachea

The unique feature I observed is the delicate balance and timing between the two structures that allow the lifesaving epiglottis to close safely and securely every time. As the swallow is initiated in the mouth and the oropharynx closes in the back of the mouth, the larynx or voice box raises the opening of the trachea (the glottis) to enable the back of the tongue to push back on the epiglottis to seal off the windpipe. This action assures the proper direction of liquid and food to the esophagus and not the trachea.

The tongue also plays a critical role at various stages in the swallow process, especially in moving the bolus and closing the epiglottis upon completion of the mission.

I started to consider whether there was some evolutionary factor that had created such a vulnerable, even life-threatening, function. I found that the head-and-neck surgeon, Terence M. Davidson, MD, had recently written an article investigating the phenomenon called obstructive sleep apnea (OSA). He was making a strong case for the cause of this condition, a serious disorder where breathing repeatedly stops and starts during sleep. The cause, Davidson noted, was relaxed muscle tone in the head and neck that can temporarily occlude the airway. OSA can be a life-threatening condition; at a minimum, it can severely affect the quality of sleep and create snoring.

Davidson further theorized about the source of this problem as dating to some major evolutionary changes in the human upper respiratory tract that occurred about forty thousand years ago. This change is unique to the human animal, and not found in any other mammal (with the curious exception of the English bulldog). He borrowed the term "great leap forward" from the evolutionary biologist Jared Diamond, PhD, who had coined it earlier to describe a dramatic shift at the time in the human bone structure in the very area of my interest: the mouth, neck, and entire head. In essence, during this time in history, many human bones underwent a shift in size, location, angle of intersection, and other ways, influencing the development and functions of the mouth, throat, and the brain.

This process, Davidson went on to explain, created some unique problems for humans, anatomically speaking. First, it caused the tongue to move back into the pharynx, with the result that the pharynx, and in turn the larynx, dropped in the throat, thereby extending the distance or gap between the epiglottis and soft palate. This meant that the so-called "soft palate lock" that all other animals possess throughout their lives, the lock that prevents big problems with coordination of swallowing and breathing, was lost for all humans.

So what was this shift all about? Davidson hypothesized that it took place as a result of the emergence of sophisticated human speech, the formation of sounds that required a different oral cavity structure. The same evolution that enabled sophisticated communication also helped in other ways, notably walking, balance, and vision; unfortunately, it created a defect that made for obstructive sleep apnea. By having kept the trachea properly closed off for all previous human history, it had been a lifesaving preventer of trouble during eating and swallowing. Now this insurance was gone.

However, it turns out that this loss of function is actually not present at birth. Only as the human infant learns to sit up does the larynx begin to fall—and that function becomes lost. This loss begins to occur at about two to six months; by age five, we have fully lost that connection. During infancy, the primary benefit of the lock is that the infant can both feed and swallow while breathing, just like all other mammals. As the infant suckles, the fluid is directed around this obstruction from the oral cavity to the pharynx.

I was drawn back to what I discussed in the previous chapter. I was thinking first of the differences I described between the swallow patterns of breast-feeding and bottle-feeding, and the effect of the difference on the development of healthy vagal tone. I also thought about how parenting factors influence healthy development of a secure attachment bond during infancy. I wondered how these two factors might affect and be affected by swallow patterns shaped in the initial years of life—by infant-feeding method, the infant's perception of security, or both. Given these three activities, breast-feeding, psychological parenting, and swallowing, what was the web of cause and effect among them?

Clearly, my questions were quite complex, and they remained only partially illuminated. The science for each was there in some coherent form. I have presented the feeding and psychology pieces in the previous chapter and the swallow pattern here. I sought—and continued to seek—the exact nature of the linkage among functions. Does the tone of the vagus nerve associated with swallowing bear a stamp, a neural sensory, and response imprint that continues so powerfully in adulthood as to unconsciously drive the quality of the swallow and the emotions triggered by the process? Doesn't the unique structure and function of the human epiglottis in the swallow pattern offer a special key to understanding? How does its function influence how information is processed and interpreted, how human decisions are made, how well decisions are made, and how well healthy self-regulation takes place?

I returned to the anatomy and physiology of the swallow pattern. I kept imagining the preverbal infant, completely dependent upon its feeding caregiver, deriving security and sustenance as it sucks and swallows. During the process, the infant unconsciously develops the neurological connections between the oral cavity and the brain. New "memories" and associative recordings in the nervous system—and vagal tone—are evaluated and recorded. It seems hard not to speculate that critical life-shaping patterns of behavior—the signature responses to life that create tooth sense—are being put in place during the first several years of life.

8

A NEW BIG PICTURE OF
HUMAN SOCIAL BEHAVIOR

This was a difficult time for me. I wasn't quite sure where to look next. I subscribed to online professional scientific research databases. I scoured the Internet, which at the time was rapidly becoming a massive source of information, albeit often of uneven quality or reliability. I shared my quest with just about anyone I knew, regardless of professional expertise, life station, or extent of life experience.

I often didn't know exactly what I was looking for. All I knew was that I wanted to help make dentistry a safe and ordinary event for my patients, not something perceived as a unique threat requiring sweat or dread. I wanted to have my patients' trust and to be fully engaged with them during appointments. The participants in this event—the patient, my assistants, and me—were humans. We had respective roles during treatment, but I wanted us to work in psychological sync. I started viewing a dental appointment as a human relationship event as much as a technical mission.

I kept telling myself not to expect too much. My work involves a special intimacy; dental treatment involves an invasion of an especially sensitive and central part of the person's neurological and physical being. The oral cavity is not just a place where a person chews, smiles, tastes, breathes, and swallows. It is the seat of unique and complex processes. It is the portal through which must pass everything physical that is needed to sustain life itself.

I reminded myself that, unlike other surgical procedures, dentistry is usually performed while the patient is awake. Granted, there is the option of general anesthesia, but it is not standard protocol and not the first choice for almost all dental procedures. Still, when most procedures of a similar order and risk are done by a medical professional on another part of the body, the patient is often given general anesthesia. Since the surgeon's solution was not really one of my options, I was definitely managing my expectations for anything new or significant.

Then, several years ago, I had a very pleasant surprise. I came across a paper that did not deal specifically with the oral cavity that jumped out at me. Written by the University of Illinois-Chicago researcher Stephen Porges, PhD, it was titled *Neuroception: A Subconscious System for Detecting Threats and Safety.* It explored, from a theoretical perspective, how a specific part of the nervous system plays a role in how we evaluate and respond to risk. The model essentially pairs how our physiological and psychological selves are affected by risks as they are perceived from the outside environment. The paper addressed how the uniqueness of each person means that each person processes experiences differently; each person has a signature response. He identified this neural function as "neuroception."

This paper is quite detailed in its presentation of neuroception. Here is a short and simplified review.

Looking at the human autonomic nervous system (ANS), Porges begins by offering two very distinct versions of how it works. The first is what is commonly understood since its identification nearly

150 years ago, and which I have mentioned in my discussion of the vagus nerve in chapter 6. The second is what is proposed and researched by Porges and his associates.

First, let me expand on the generally received understanding—the one I was taught in dental school in the 1980s. The ANS is inextricably connected with regulating our responses to what we experience. It evolved in our ancestors many millennia ago, and it has served to keep us alive by making us choose appropriate responses to potentially threatening situations. It scans everything out there as either dangerous or safe. The ANS works under the radar, though, underneath our level of consciousness; it senses and responds automatically by triggering the action of our organs. The ANS consists of two branches: the parasympathetic generates a rest-and-rebuild response, and the sympathetic generates the fight-or-flight response. Also, the ANS, though best known for its regulatory function while we are under stress or calm, is also largely responsible for control of the more mundane functions of the body (breathing, heartbeat, and digestion).

This is how the story has gone—and how it still goes in much of the scientific community. Since it was standard understanding in academia, the understanding has been held without much question by most of the dental profession until now. It's what we all have learned in school. It's almost as much a part of the received science as the theory of evolution itself. And, most critically, it's the universal basis for dental treatment decisions based by consensus on assumed scientific accuracy, adequacy, and applicability.

So now enter the second version of how the ANS functions, the Porges version. As noted, the version when presented was the culmination of at least twenty years of research by Porges and his colleagues. In effect, it was breaking new ground by describing a model of the ANS that included, not just the two branches (sympathetic and parasympathetic), but a distinct third branch, which he identified as the social nervous system. To identify this system, he interchangeably uses "the social engagement system." He postulates a much larger role for the vagus nerve than the one already premised in other work by breast-feeding researchers and others. Porges goes further, proposing and documenting that its unique evolution in humans makes it a key player in human social life—and how we act in social situations. He looks at how the vagus exerts a mediating effect on different organ systems, an effect that complements the two inherited branches, especially the parasympathetic, and potentiates human capacity for engaging with one another in ways that we term "human." We are more connected on an emotional and psychological level—more rational—than is possible for other animals.

He has called his theory the polyvagal theory. It is very complex, but suffice it to say that the "poly" in "polyvagal" refers to the unique way in which two particular fibers of the vagus nerve evolved separately over time and how the resulting third branch of the ANS was accompanied by a huge evolutionary shift in the behavioral nature of our species.

Neurologically speaking, the polyvagal theory postulates that humans do not simply have two branches of the autonomic nervous system, acting in a reciprocal off-on way to manage self-regulation. According to Porges, there are three neurologically sequenced branches; the branches operate sequentially instead of reciprocally.

In this model, the social engagement system is first in line, and it is what is at work in social situations. These specific situations involve any perception of verbal and nonverbal cues from other people. Taking cues from such signals as facial expression, tone of voice, and body language, this system reads, decodes, responds, and directs the way a person engages with others.

Precision and accuracy in reading the threat potential of any social situation is critical to the social engagement system in fulfilling its role or course. There is much involved both neurologically and psychologically in each person's unique past that can serve to abet or hinder how well this third system functions. For now, simply keep in mind that Porges considers this system unique to humans. This "first-responder" capability is in effect what makes us human. It enables our full potential of experiencing and expressing what it is to be alive and connected, making accurate risk assessments and appropriate decisions in a social context, not just for mere survival. It makes civilized society possible.

When the social engagement system is overwhelmed by the sense of threat, the second system in line—the sympathetic—takes over and mobilizes a self-protective high alert mode. This is manifested in many physical ways, such as faster respiration and quicker pulse, and typically is experienced emotionally in its extreme manifestation as anxiety or panic.

If the polyvagal and sympathetic systems are overwhelmed by perceived immediate danger, the parasympathetic steps in to keep us alive by causing us to freeze. This mode is characterized by slower breath and heart rate and experienced emotionally as a letting go or dissociation. This is the last line of resort in the face of perceived imminent annihilation; it is designed to make you feel your very presence disappear, so to speak.

Porges also states that, on a conscious level, humans can hardly be aware of any of this happening. This is not the work of the prefrontal cortex part of the brain, where conscious thinking and decision making takes place. The sequencing is essentially instantaneous. There are no committee meetings, but the process is essential to enabling survival at the optimal level under any given circumstances.

I became very excited to learn more about neuroception and how to make practical use of its principles. With a greater appreciation of the workings of the autonomic nervous system, I thought, I might be able to interpret and respond to patient behavior with more precision. Perhaps I could devise specific steps to take when I saw certain shifts in the engagement level of patients during treatment. Perhaps I could keep them, in Porges's terms, "socially engaged" rather than "sympathetically" hyperalert and reactive while I went about my work. I was surprised and challenged by what happened.

9

BUT DENTISTRY IS DIFFERENT

As I began to go about looking for ways to use the concepts of neuroception in helping patients deal with the stress of treatment, I did not consider myself naive about the challenge and prospects for success. I reminded myself that dentistry, when provided without a sedative, creates a perfect opportunity for stress. I would need to become especially observant and astute in detecting and responding to verbal and nonverbal cues to help anxious patients remain "socially engaged." Knowing that the patient's ability to remain socially engaged may be compromised with either real or perceived potential pain events always just around the corner, it would clearly be challenging to make social interventions (through my words, gestures, movements, tone of voice, facial expression, management of the environment—in any number of ways) in order to minimize the chances that a patient would default to a sympathetic fight-or-flight state—regardless of my good intentions, sensitivity, or commitment to maintain trust.

But I was still hopeful. I was determined to try what I could. I tried to refine various strategies—some of which I had already been using, even though all were based on my admittedly incomplete understanding of neuroception. I did this with what I saw later was incomplete awareness of the risk: that my good intentions might not always be appreciated, especially by patients more accustomed to stoicism and "getting on with it." Patients might have the opposite reaction. This could be a slippery slope.

I initially started carving out a few moments before each appointment with patients whose profile and past history might put me on alert. I would consciously check the state of my own "social engagement system" to prepare myself for creating the relational aspect of the care I was about to provide. I noted the patient who was waiting and reminded myself that I was not just dealing with dental issues—but with supporting how that person might tolerate care and manage a response. For me, this usually amounted to taking a few deep breaths and slowing down for a moment. Within the course of a busy day, I thought this might allow me to feel clearer and be fully present for the next patient who was to be treated.

For example, if I sensed or noticed something shifting in the patient's position or facial expression during preparation for an injection, I would use specifically tailored, even rehearsed engaging words, mirroring to the patient what I heard and also noting with a neutral tone what I was observing with him or her. While injecting, I might say softly, "I'm going slowly so that it will be better absorbed and be more comfortable." I would observe whether the patient took my cues to relax. If he or she did not, and I noticed any forced or irregular breathing, tight fists, or sweat beads, I might offer additional supportive words, affirmations, supply a breathing tip or exercise, or ask him or her to visualize light of a certain color within a certain region of his or her body.

I saw the positive effect that these tools had on the highly charged emotional state of some patients. They definitely helped— but not always and not predictably. Different patients responded differently to different modulating tools. Some responded favorably to a particular approach; others resisted the very same thing. I was glad to have several methods to help patients who gravitated and instinctively reacted more favorably to tools designed to tap into the sense of sound, vision, or touch. At times I was astonished by how rigid and unyielding some patients' responses were to my suggestions.

It was especially interesting to see whether a patient's reaction differed depending on whether what I was doing was discomforting or not. Even when I was working in an area where there was no real possibility of my causing pain—maybe checking if the grooves of back teeth that were free of decay—patients who were hypervigilant would brace and grimace as if there was actual pain. The imagined prospect, not based on the reality of the moment, caused the reaction. If this automatic bracing occurred regardless, then what if anything could I or anyone do to modify that perception?

There were also practical considerations. Even if my approach to communication and the relational component of dentistry had enormous potential and was guided by good intentions, what I could offer was dictated by my schedule. The opportunity to engage as I have described was really within a relatively brief window. I never felt I could be completely present for more than a certain period of time; I always had an eye on the clock. This was not conducive to complete relaxation and safety. The schedule created an urgency to engage within a set period of time—and then move in regardless of where we were to finish the job and get on to the next patient. I must admit that one patient's issues blended into another, and I was challenged to track individual situations accurately.

This pressure to deliver the right response interfered with my own self-regulation. I would often find myself jumping in more quickly than was best, acting on some hasty inference or even hoping that what had worked with another patient would work in the present situation. I sometimes made too quick an intuitive leap. Or worse, I made the mistake of telling them what they were failing to do—as if I knew better or more than they did—instead of listening. Sometimes I was giving orders rather than making suggestions. I rationalized all this with my need to keep to the schedule.

In retrospect, I see that there is a fine line in using suggestions rather than a more assertive approach to intercede in the coping process. This lapse gave me insight into the bigger issue; dentistry is different. Trying to make the neuroception model apply to the practice of dentistry was like trying to fit the proverbial square peg into the round hole. The success of the process was very much about what I brought to the moment in terms of my mental and emotional state.

I often wondered if what I was doing was worth the effort. Was I working harder than my patients? They probably had no idea about what I was experiencing internally; for all I knew, that was the last thing on their minds.

The need to address the behavior that I had been initially trained to ignore did not go away. The neuroception theory did not include a manual for applying it, and it was disappointingly inadequate for my purposes. I could not simply turn back the clock and revert to seeing myself as a technician providing customer service. I was stuck even further with my dissatisfaction at such an acceptable prospect.

Ultimately, it came back to square one. My patients were people first, and this basic understanding had to come first. I was working in the home territory of my patients' core vulnerable structures. This was not all about me and my performance and corrective actions, implementing a technique.

For anxious patients, the bottom line about my mission was that my work and I were not welcome. No matter how hard I tried, my techniques and I could not transcend the unconscious and conscious danger signals that went off in this uniquely sensitive area of the human body. This is what happens when dentists set about their work with patients in distress. There is no tactical way to avoid it.

By coming to appreciate the complexity of what might be transpiring in another person's experience, I was undergoing a sea change in perspective. The perfectionist in me was coming to see that it was not a matter of getting everything exactly right in the human interaction. There simply wasn't any such thing as "perfectly right," and that if only from exhaustion I needed to let go, regardless of my disappointment. It was as if I had been hit square between the eyes. I decided to be a close observer of the treatment process and of myself, more cautious about my assumptions and attempts to manage situations. I found myself becoming less impelled to get the exactly correct intervention while I was performing a procedure. It was a fool's errand. No pun intended, but this understanding was making me more "patient."

Fortunately, the process of becoming more empathic and understanding of my patient's vulnerabilities—and of being self-forgiving—gave me fresh energy and perspective. It renewed my excitement to stay with my project, albeit with fewer expectations. I reminded myself that this was, in the familiar saying, a journey, not a destination. Although I might not find big "answers," the neurological activity I was calling "tooth sense" was an activity or force whose subtleties and implications deserved more detective work.

My concept certainly included accepting the generic validity of neuroception theory, but it only partially provided an explanation for the unique subtleties of the oral cavity and swallowing pattern at work. It was certainly not a set of operating instructions for individual situations. The nervous system evaluates social situations in a way unique to humans and is unavailable to other species.

Thinking of dentistry as a major "social situation" is very important, but how the quality of one's neuroception actually modulated or was modulated by the nature of the whole structure and function of the region, especially the epiglottis and the swallowing pattern, was not clear or even subject to explanation.

Yes, it was clear that vagal tone in general could very well predispose all dental patients to outsized sensitivity and vulnerability, some more so than others. Yes, individual biology and biography made things easier or more difficult for any given patient. But whatever my questions, answered or not, now I needed simply to adjust my perspective toward them and my patients accordingly.

10

COMING TO MY SENSES

As I came to terms with acknowledging my unrealistic expectations that the concept of neuroception was not going to transform treatment strategies, it struck me that I had been distracted in my quest from the much wider picture of perception. Neuroception had been "a bright, shiny object." I was fascinated, but it was not the only object in the display case. The brain receives and responds to sensation in many ways. The working of the vagus nerve does matter in the larger schematic of tooth sense, but it suggested another aspect of tooth sense. There was no practical or accurate in-the-moment application during a dental procedure that could reliably make a difference in how the patient experienced what was happening.

What about the role of other ways of sensing? I became curious about a whole other class of ways of perception that I had previously overlooked or discounted. An investigation into internal senses took me to reviewing from a different angle what occurs when we sense what is happening to us—not from the outside (what we hear, see, touch, taste, or smell), but from our insides. In addition to these five external senses, we have at least five internal senses that give us information about our inner states.

These five internal senses are important: thermoception (temperature sense), equilibrioception (sense of balance), kinesthesioception (sense of speed of movement or acceleration), nociception (sense of pain), and perhaps most important of all, proprioception (sense of location or position). These senses give us an awareness of our selves, of our internal states.

Senses

← External Senses →
Tactile (Touch)
Visual (Sight)
Auditory (Hearing)
Gustatory (Taste)
Olfactory (Smell)

→ Internal Senses ←
Equilibrioception (Balance)
Thermoception (Temperature)
Nociception (Pain)
Kinesthesioception (Acceleration)
Proprioception (Position)

In general, these internal senses do not work in isolation or independent of one another. They all rely on associated nerve fibers that relay information to the brain. Each does its job by responding to position, speed and acceleration, temperature, balance, or pain (or degree of comfort or discomfort). When I reach for a hot mug, I am relying on several internal senses: my sense of position to keep me from missing the handle, my sense of temperature and pain from burning myself if I spill hot contents, and my sense of balance from spilling the contents or perhaps pitching flat on my face when I reach for the cup.

With regard to the workings of internal senses in the oral environment, proprioception and nociception are the most noteworthy. Their unique functions and connection in the oral cavity may have the effect of amplifying patient anxiety.

The proprioceptive fibers convey information regarding the body's position precisely and moment by moment, telling you whether you are standing, sitting, or reclining. They track an awareness of how your limbs move through space and where they are located in relation to everything in your environment. This sense is much nuanced; it precisely communicates speed, angle, and balance. Along with equilibrioception, it keeps you from falling or bumping into anything and keeps you at the appropriate distance from things.

As for nociception, the associated fibers convey a sense of pain. These fibers work in tandem with proprioceptive fibers to help you respond instantly to a perceived threat to your physical well-being. These fibers locate pain or discomfort precisely. If you receive an insect bite or sting, for example, you not only feel the pain, you can sense precisely where it is coming from. The pain instantaneously draws your attention while the position sense allows you to respond appropriately. It is there to help keep you alive, safe, and protected in an emergency; it guides attention to the source. In this sense, pain is a good thing. However, in the process, it activates the sympathetic nervous system and challenges a person's self-regulation. That is why it is hard to feel pain and relax at the same time.

What it is curious about the interaction of these two senses with regard to teeth is that teeth, unlike the rest of your anatomical structures, do not have proprioceptive fibers. The socket that holds the teeth and the jaw joint has them—but teeth do not. Consequently, teeth are not good at relaying feedback about position or locating the source of a pain, such as certain types of toothaches. Experiencing pain without knowing exactly where it is coming from may account for increasing anxiety. Even without any pain being sensed—with dental work that does not involve work that does not produce pain or when a patient has been anesthetized—this potential anxiety still exists.

To illustrate further, let's compare a patient receiving a dental filling with one receiving stitches on the hand. With both, our modern health-care system uses Novocain to anesthetize the local area. In both cases, there is a potential for anxiety because of the perceived threat of some impending insult to the body. It is inescapable—the sense is that it has to happen, and it has to happen right now!

However, the situations have significant differences. In the case of the stitching process, the patient can see what is going on; the dental patient can't. That alone is cause for the dental patient to be more anxious. But more subtly, the sensory systems at work in the two locations operate very differently. Both signal where the action is occurring (proprioception), but the system in the mouth provides both a stronger signal of pain (nociception) and also a less precise signal. The hand's proprioceptive fibers relay position very precisely, enabling the patient to accurately assess the situation and to self-soothe or self-regulate more. The proprioceptive fibers in the teeth, on the other hand, do not convey location as accurately and thus make the patient more vulnerable and challenged to manage emotional reaction. For the dental patient, the combined effect of strong pain sensation, inability to see what is happening, and also inability to sense exactly where the pain is coming from all add up to a much more potentially challenging and distressing situation than the one faced by the patient whose hand is being stitched.

If this combination of factors were not enough, here is also another noteworthy difference between receiving stitches and having a tooth filled. Many dentists lean the patient back to a supine position. The external sense of hearing decreases when one is lying down. Being in that position in an environment with jumbled, unpleasant noises, muffled conversation, and miscellaneous ambient sound can easily make dependence on the internal senses for assessing the relative safety or danger of the situation the best, though imperfect, option for the patient.

Incidentally, the anxiety over the lack of position sense doesn't necessarily require the patient to be present in the dental office for treatment. I see this frequently with a toothache that is reported as causing discomfort but not unbearable pain. Patients call in, needing immediate treatment for what they describe as a toothache. When asked for specifics, they often cannot clearly identify the problem area. Even when these patients come into the office and are in the chair, they are still often not able to differentiate which tooth in the quadrant, or quarter of the mouth, is the source. Sometimes they cannot even say for sure which quadrant the pain is coming from—or whether it originates in the top or bottom jaw.

Ironically, the absence of precise position sense in the tooth may well have an upside. It might be very distracting if, while eating, we were to get as many as thirty-two simultaneously different sets of feedback at once concerning the bolus our teeth are negotiating. Pardon the pun, but this would be a lot to chew on.

However, as I write now, my curiosity leaves me feeling that there must be some additional proprioceptive functions that compensate for this lack of tooth position sense. I would like to explore that more fully, but it might take up a whole other book to accomplish it. What is important and germane to this particular book is how these individual observations and scientific understanding of this terrain affect care. That is the job of the next chapter.

I have not included this discussion because it is necessarily helpful or applicable to how treatment is administered. It probably isn't. And it does not take us further in exploring the nuances of tooth sense. Proprioception, like all the other internal "ceptions," works the same way for everyone. But I include it here simply as general information whose possession might still serve to reduce the fear and anxiety that occur without it.

There's one other reason I have included it. Though this information does not address the issue of individual differences in the quality of tooth sense, it has opened room for me to do so at some further future point. That study project involves returning to an examination of the role of the vagus nerve and its involvement in the workings of the internal senses. I'm still looking to elucidate the neurological action involved in swallowing. The impulse or need to swallow can be very unpleasant. I see the discomfort every day. I want to understand why some patients do better than others at managing dentistry, including swallowing during treatment.

Creating a hypothesis would involve taking a closer look at how the swallowing patterns we acquire from infancy affect vagal tone, one's ability in later life to adapt and respond, and how I might use such understanding to further improve my patients' experience of dentistry.

So I really want to bring things full circle, but my hunches and inferences are still on the drawing board and will wait to be fully explored.

While this project has still been awaiting progress, I recently had a rich, impactful experience that actually did not explicitly involve proprioception but was so compelling that I tell about it here as a fitting way to bring this narrative to its conclusion.

11

TOOTH SENSE—
REACHING BEYOND SCIENCE

This story involves a very memorable patient visit. Whether this was just the right moment waiting for something big or small to happen, I have no way of knowing. It really doesn't matter. It seems a fitting way to end this book, illustrating that, beyond any relevant science, dentistry is a relationship event.

The dental patient gives up control of the situation for an hour or more. From a psychological standpoint, power has been given to me and my team. In my dental training, no one would think about discussing the powerlessness a patient might feel. That was for the mental health specialists. Yet this is quite often the proverbial elephant in the living room. This subject has been off-limits—not to be brought up or considered. Successful dentistry involves carefully avoiding, rather than acknowledging, the patient's vulnerability and coping challenges. It's a surgical matter. Like many of my colleagues, I frequently let the "elephant" dominate the situation.

For many patients, the psychology of giving up power and putting trust in the professional is not an issue. Nothing is triggered. However, it is present for many patients. Although this sense of powerlessness is clearly reflected in patients who do not (or cannot) hide discomfort or anxiety, it can be a factor for patients who seem calm and easygoing. Patients who come socially engaged and interactive may, as if turning on a dime, start to resist as the treatment proceeds.

Regardless of a patient's initial demeanor, when there is resistance to surrendering to the work at hand, I usually see it first in body language, specifically in mouths. Patients may open their mouths minimally, limiting access for the work at hand, even though I might gently and continuously request that they open wider. Sometimes patients will turn to the opposite side I am working on, as if they are pulling away. Their cheeks might become taut—or they will contract their tongue with all their might—while the rest of the body may be relaxed and seemingly disconnected from the contortions occurring from the neck up. The patient may also be rigid, frozen, or fidgeting to the point of writhing.

A longtime patient I'll call Sarah usually did a good job of self-regulation when we began treatment. Then she would quite abruptly become agitated. This time was no different.

At the outset, an observer would not have noticed anything unusual. Sarah came in acting very upbeat. We had a conversation about her children's summer activities. When we started to talk about the procedure for the day, she became noticeably quieter. Although Sarah was socially engaged when talking about sports camps or describing how she was looking forward to a week at the Jersey Shore with her family, when it came time to start the work, she became remarkably timid. She began fidgeting and kept adjusting her position in the chair.

As I was about to begin the procedure, she became completely quiet. When I asked basic questions, such as whether she would like a pillow for extra support, she was barely able to manage a meek nod. At one point, she began moving her head quickly to her right as if she was responding to my movement—even though I had not yet begun.

Thinking of Stephen Porges and imagining Sarah's neuroception process at work, I saw her social engagement system defaulting to the danger warning of her sympathetic system. If verbalized, they might have said, "What is this guy doing to me with all this stuff?!" Her cheek became taut, and she opened up only about halfway. Her breathing became forced and shallow.

I continued with the preparation and slowly gave her Novocain on the part of her gum called the lower dental arch. Suddenly, her body started sliding around in the dental chair. Although Sarah's abrupt turn in behavior was what I had come to expect, something stopped me from what I was doing to make things more comfortable. I found myself seeing her behavior differently. I sat Sarah up in the chair, and said, "Sarah, I can see that you're uncomfortable."

Rather than proceeding, I waited for a response. She nodded.

I said, "You may think that all of this is being thrust upon you—and that you are powerless in what is happening to you. Is that what is happening? Does that make sense to you?"

Again, she nodded meekly, and said simply, "I don't like all this stuff."

I said, "Thank you for sharing that. Your honesty and openness are the keys to your comfort. I want you to be as comfortable as you can, but I can only help to the level that you allow me to. This is a two-way street, and we are both part of a team."

I paused to check if this made sense to her. Again she nodded.

I continued, "It is really important to me that you to understand that you actually do hold the power as to how you choose to respond here. Understanding your power to choose your response is as important for a successful outcome as is the technical part of care. I can help you with that. How does that sound to you?"

She nodded again.

I didn't feel that I had really gotten through or changed anything in her perspective. Instead of proceeding as I would ordinarily, I waited. Her rapid breathing and fixed stare made we waver and almost abandon my small experiment. I didn't want to cause further anxiety through delay, and that was a large tug for me. *Get back to your work. Get on with it! She doesn't want to prolong the agony!* Something made me pause.

At that moment, my dental assistant Kristen saw this pregnant pause too. Somewhat unexpectedly, she stepped in and said, "Sarah? How does what Dr. Oras just mentioned make you feel?"

There was a pause. Again she just nodded, but there seemed to be even less energy in her response.

Part of me wanted to take Kristen out of the equation and disregard her involvement. I was in control, after all. I decided to wait and let her continue. There was risk here—but also opportunity. I knew Sarah quite well and was counting on enough trust to proceed.

Kristen said, "It is important for you to feel that any emotions and feelings you are experiencing are valuable and necessary for you, Sarah. Don't quench the light inside of you that is giving energy to your power."

Once more, she nodded.

Wow! This is interesting. My assistant is onto something.

I held back as she continued, slowly and with pauses.

"We are here to help make this easy for you, but it's not only in our hands. You control all of the cards here. Do you believe that?"

She nodded more emphatically.

"It's understandable that you are probably thinking and feeling that you are having all this thrust upon you, and that you are not in control. But, Sarah, you are most definitely in control. You can decide whether this treatment is to go along easily or not." She paused, waiting for her to acknowledge her words and to make sure she had her permission to keep going.

What was remarkable was that, through it all, she did not say anything. However, in what was probably only three minutes, a shift occurred in Sarah's energy and inner perspective. Her body contortion disappeared as she relaxed quietly in the chair. Her cheek lost its tautness. Her breathing became deeper and normal. She smiled, slightly, but it was still a smile. She had taken on a calm demeanor.

Kristen—and then I—asked if she was ready to proceed. She nodded one final time—emphatically. Her nods seemed more and more confident and emphatic.

So though the treatment that followed was in itself neither more nor less inherently uncomfortable than what I had always provided Sarah, what was markedly different was the quality of her response. Something had happened to make it possible, and I was interested in knowing what helped her turn the corner with her own "neuroception" in the moment! As we finished, and everything had been removed from her mouth, I wondered if she would at last verbalize and perhaps even debrief us about what had happened.

I wondered whether I would hear the first version of Sarah, full of banter about her upcoming vacation and some upbeat, maybe even witty comment. But what I got instead was a version of Sarah that I hadn't seen before. She was noticeably lighter, relaxed with what appeared to be a deeper sense of self. She slowly and purposefully gave me an extended look in the eye and a firm handshake. "Thanks for everything," she said, walking to the front desk.

Allowing an element I had been trained to ignore, avoid, or somehow "take out," had become the fulcrum for something more than successful treatment. It had seemed to allow for the healthy restoration of my patient's social engagement after I had missed the mark with so many previous attempts. I had often seen palpable, reinforced evidence that whatever we think or have heard about dental care—the good, bad, or the ugly—we are not inextricably trapped into believing in the "truth," an experience that our mind might conjure up. Yes, some aspects of tooth sense dictated the neurological term—but not the perspective that could be taken with the right human connection. Achieving success could be easy if the treatment team and the patient together could find an elegant yet relaxed path.

That event with Sarah was a defining moment for me. It involved risk. For me, it was the risk of holding back for a minute or two to see if some richer dimension could be brought to bear without making things more complicated—and the risk of letting go of the whole procedure before Kristen's beautiful intervention. I would never have thought of doing anything like that in my dental assistant days. This was a sharing of the power.

For Kristen, as I discovered later, it was the risk of upsetting the flow of events as prescribed by usual protocol. She could have been reprimanded for an unwelcome intrusion. For Sarah, it was the biggest risk of all: trusting that she could safely exercise her power to regulate her own anxiety, even when that involved willingly giving the power to others. Together, with our support, she had been able to turn vulnerability into an asset—no small doing. That was, I'm imagining, a substantial takeaway for her.

As an afterthought, I recently came across a description of a form of the Asian martial art called Aikido. Aikido practice involves using and relating to the energy of another person so as to move the potential synergy between the two of you in a positive and collaborative direction. The guiding maxim is: *When pushed, you pull; when pulled, you push. You find the natural course and bend with it.* This maxim seemed to encapsulate what I have come to terms with in working relationally with patients. It is, after all, another aspect of tooth sense—albeit not one to be dissected or understood better by scientific inquiry.

12

AN UNFINISHED QUEST

There are no doubt many for whom my personal story and professional odyssey is of only passing interest. Many patients and dentists have not experienced dissatisfaction with the way things are done in dentistry. I have many such patients, and that's fine. I am not seeking to stir up dissatisfaction where none exists! But I wouldn't have written this book had I not seen so many patients who are dissatisfied with how they deal with dentistry—or how dentistry deals with them. Having been frustrated by the shortcomings, I have been challenged by my own resourcefulness in responding in those situations.

I have shared parts of my life story as a preamble to my quest, which though professional, has never been without a prominent and powerful complementary personal dimension. It seems serendipitous that I would have the opportunity to come to piece together this scientific puzzle this way. I was at loss to effectively self-regulate during the emotionally charged events of my childhood. As with just about all of us growing up at that time, my parents did the very best they could to raise their children with the best precepts and examples they knew. Whatever I missed out on was in no way their intentional doing. They operated with the information and ideas available to them. Neuroscience and human development theory at the time was itself in its infancy and what was known was not widely disseminated. I can see clearly now that they had to rely on—and were responding to—what they had absorbed either consciously or unconsciously in their own lives.

I believe the deficiencies I experienced have turned out to be the source of my passion and strength. This passion has expressed and manifested itself in two complementary ways. First, it has impelled me to get a rational grasp of why there exists the unique involvement of dentistry, the oral cavity, and tooth sense in the shaping of individual behavior, thought, and feeling. It also made me more empathic and disposed to acknowledging the role of intuition, and to finding ways not simply to "feel the pain" of others, but to ameliorate my patients' experiences with dentistry.

It is ironic that I—who has not actually experienced much dentistry as a patient—would be writing a book to address the emotional concerns of those who have. I came to believe I could do so because the events of my childhood, though not apparently related, seemed to correlate on an emotional level with what I have continually seen and imagined going on with my own patients. I do not know the intimate details or the full biography of my patients. When I perceive the buttoned-up stoicism of a patient about to experience a potentially uncomfortable procedure, I can instantly connect through my own experiences with my father at the dinner table.

I can also relate to patients who react to treatment in the opposite way. Such situations invariably bring to mind the conversation with my father and friends in our driveway. As with Sarah, I overreacted to an emotionally charged situation by mistakenly assuming it was up to me to make everything go well. I lacked trust in others to work it out. I almost absurdly tried to control the conversation and flow of events that really were not about me or for me to manage. In my confusion, I missed the cues that could have evoked a much more appropriate and rational response.

When my patients exhibit comparable behavior, I can readily put myself in their emotional shoes. In doing so, I can be more empathetic with the patients' situation and feelings. I not only see the neuroscience and inadequate tooth sense aspects of the patients' reaction on a rational level—I can connect to their feelings of being overwhelmed and powerless.

Returning to the scientific aspect of my quest, I have noted and tracked how it led to speculation and then gradual clarification of the concept of tooth sense as an explanation-in-progress of the relationship between certain neurological, psychological, and sociological components of behavior. These components are uniquely activated during dentistry, mainly because they are connected with the biology and the biography of each person's oral cavity. This book carries an invitation to fellow dentists, professional and amateur scientists, those thinking outside and beyond science, and anyone curious about the subject to become co-participants in this quest.

I described how I could not find satisfactory answers to my questions and concerns about care through streamlined management methods of office layout or the newest implements and procedures. Everything in that domain seemed to deal mostly with the externals of care, such as new technology or office arrangement. I have dutifully kept current on technology and protocols, and at I even came close to implementing the *Front Desklessness* model proposed by Dr. Dickerson. What was missing in such pursuit was a perspective on dentistry that acknowledged the whole cast of players during treatment—the patient, the staff, and I—were first of all human beings dealing with an unnatural and invasive activity. The entire process needed to be based on full, open psychological engagement rather than avoidance or denial.

Stephen Porges's scientifically promising new paradigm of human social behavior revisited traditional depictions of neurological processes. It gave me hope for a better understanding of what I felt was a core missing piece to dental care. However, I came to be only partially satisfied with the polyvagal theory and the idea of neuroception as a comprehensive paradigm for explaining the unique elements of dentistry and, more importantly, for providing any practical guide for my team and me.

I began looking more closely at actual structures and operations of the mouth as the next step in my search. I looked at the special neurological sensitivities required of all the components of the oral cavity as they work together to produce the swallow—and how the legacy of human evolution and the individual's own early life experiences shape the nature of response to the dramatic situation that unfolds for each patient upon entering the treatment room and taking a seat in the chair. This search yielded a much more practical and respectful way to approach treating patients, as well as a wider curiosity about how these structures and their workings might influence the signature response to life for all of us.

Most recently, what seems like a natural progression toward acknowledging and appreciating the role of intuition and empathy in creating a patient's safety and complete self-regulation has given me the final push to complete what I could and also accept that it's a work in progress.

What follows is a thumbnail summary of my thoughts about what is now in the offing for further consideration. In the resources section that follows the conclusion, I have placed further notes on some of these references for those who wish to explore further.

First, I'm interested in other possible functions that these vulnerable structures may serve in infant development beyond shaping vagal tone. Both current research and common sense suggest that achieving a secure attachment bond of infant to mother along with breast-feeding, create an optimal path to healthy child development. Yet it would seem to me that there are other functioning systems as well that contribute neurologically and socially early on as well as patterns that will set the stage for the rest of the infant's life.

I want to look more broadly at the relationship between the whole nervous system and the endocrine system of glands. The endocrine system, like the nervous system, relays information throughout the body. The endocrine system functions via hormones, substances secreted directly into the bloodstream, whereas nerves like the vagus send their signals coursing along the via neurotransmitters, the electrical impulses in neurons. My interest relates to how hormones may mediate or contribute early on to creating the quality of attachment bond with the caregiver, the extent to which these patterns become embedded or memorized, and the extent to which they are amenable to conscious regulation in later life.

I also wish to consider the role of hormones in the process of dental decay—and to help my patients minimize decay's devastating effects. I came across some promising research in *Dentinal Fluid Transport* by Clyde Roggenkamp. It proposes a model for how hormonal function may determine the health or disease of a tooth. Though the book is little known, it describes forty years of research by two of the author's former teachers, Ralph Steinman, DDS, one of the founders of the Loma Linda University School of Dentistry, and his research partner and endocrinologist, John Leonora, DDS. My specific interest is not merely to consider how pertinent hormones are involved in regulating whether a tooth will decay or remain healthy and flourish. I am also curious about how this regulation process may contribute more widely to how a person might self-regulate throughout life.

I am also interested more generally in the whole field of neuroscience and the potential of new technology to explore in precise detail the operation of the entire brain as it goes about processing, storing, and responding to the continuous sensory input that we call "experience." The oral cavity where I focus my attention in work and research is only one part of the total nervous system continuously feeding and receiving responses from the brain. How the oral cavity segment of the network may affect or be affected by other components of the nervous system is the larger frame of reference I am curious about. The business of self-regulation is certainly not the exclusive domain of the oral cavity. To focus on it exclusively would be myopic.

The recent refinement of Functional Magnetic Resonance Imaging (fMRI) technology offers new ways of mapping brain activity of the brain in great detail. Much is being learned about the nuances of how the brain functions. Never before have neuroscientists been able to see precisely how areas of the brain react in real time while subjects' responses to various stimuli are tested.

This technology has also served to demystify "panic attacks" by looking at a structure of the brain called the amygdala. The amygdala stores and sorts out memories and acts as a kind of detective to alert you to danger and react quickly to what is perceived as dangerous. It records everything about an experience—even things we're not consciously taking in, such as light, shade, colors, noises, shapes, and smells. The amygdala keeps complete files and updates them continuously. This process is essential to keeping you alive. But it's not that smart—not at all. It doesn't "think." It doesn't distinguish between the past memory and the present event. It gives off false alarms—and lots of false positives!

I am curious about the limits of human capacity to consciously override the amygdala's imperative when that imperative is a false alarm, perhaps through knowing how to prepare and pre-frame the event from another perspective. In the dental treatment area, I would imagine that everyone must unconsciously go through a checklist of specific sensory elements—the chair, the voices, the equipment, opening one's mouth, even the sound of the drill. If there is an element they may not have been prepared to swallow, so to speak, or suddenness, or where the intensity has not been anticipated, the amygdala may take charge and override everything else.

What about further dimensions of the relational aspects of dentistry—and the social transactions involved? I have already made frequent mention of how my traditional training and early professional experience bypassed the relational aspects of dentistry through traditional and conventional protocols. Treating a patient's dental problem was seen as a calculated precision attack. My assistants and I were like highly trained Navy SEALS. The method of operation consists of swooping in during a precision strike, taking control over the decay that was attacking the patient, and extracting all the bad stuff so that you can save the day. "You get in and you get out," as the boss in my first practice put it, and he demonstrated it daily. Further, under his close scrutiny, any young dentist deviated at his or her peril. The mindset required for this precision work was that patient resistance was an extraneous obstacle that needed to be negotiated or removed. Such were the secret heroics of dentistry.

In my opinion, patients can be empowered and facilitated by the treatment team to take charge of their perspectives and know they have the final say—as was the case with Sarah.

This book has laid out my evolving progression in considering the behavior of patients as primarily human and not simply as dental interaction. Can a tool as sophisticated as an fMRI help offer guidance here—except as a reminder of the limitations of technology and science?

In a different vein, several researchers in the evolving branch of neuroscience seek to understand the connections between our neural hardwiring, mental health, emotion, and our genetic heritage. This field, often referred to as affective neuroscience, explores human potential and human limitation through clinical studies involving observed behaviors. They are primarily psychological or neurological.

Stumbling on Happiness by Harvard psychologist Dan Gilbert, PhD, explains why humans are so bad at being happy, specifically as it relates to valuing our future states. Daniel Goleman, PhD, in his landmark long-time bestselling book *Emotional Intelligence*, has taken up this call to explore the science of our emotions—and specifically how they influence decision making.

In *The Emotional Life of Your Brain*, Richard J. Davidson, PhD, identifies six emotional styles and posited that, unlike "personality traits," these styles actually make up our characteristic brain signature and determine how we respond or adapt to any given situation.

Sandra and Matthew Blakeslee's *The Body Has a Mind of Its Own: How Body Maps in Your Brain Help You Do (Almost) Everything Better* identifies and reports on the maps of the brain responsible for so-called interoceptive self-awareness (see chapter 10). I want to know much more about the interoceptive involvement of the teeth, mouth, and gums in relation to the overall workings of this process in the whole body.

Finally, Michael Gurian, MFA, a mental health therapist, has written prolifically about the neuroscience (as opposed to cultural influence) behind gender differences and relationship challenges that can be traced to hardwired difference in brain anatomy. One of special interest to me is *What Could He Be Thinking? How a Man's Mind Really Works*.

The paradigm of *Tooth Sense*, albeit still only partially identified and described, remains my frame of reference. The unique anatomical structure, physiological function, and psychological and emotional energy of the oral cavity continue to intrigue and fascinate me as I see my clients and respond to their diverse needs. I continue to ponder the way humans swallow and how the process requires a certain trust and letting go, a leap of emotional faith when our conscious control of organizing and preparing for this event is given over to the unconscious completion of the transaction of our digestive and assimilative organs. How is it that human evolution has somehow planted this all-or-nothing emotional event (failure could mean choking!) where it has? And how is its quality mediated by early life experience?

Although much of human perception and response is not subject to negotiation, the quest to take charge of what we can is what human life seems to be all about. For dentistry, whether this means spreading more patient education throughout the profession, becoming stronger advocates for breast-feeding and early childhood parenting education, promoting changes in dental training, or simply keeping the relational aspect at the heart of what we do, it is clearly worth the effort.

I find it ironic that the human loss of our epiglottis soft palate lock is the evolutionary culprit in making dentistry an anxious event; the profound trade-off for the loss has been our unique ability to make the precise sounds we call language—sounds also represented in writing. Being human may mean being anxious, but it gives us the chance to communicate through words to connect and evolve as no other known species can.

Ultimately, regardless of the paths of investigation that my innate curiosity takes me and my cohorts on, one principle remains clear: My practice is relationship-based. We use a specifically designed intake process to identify key features that help us draw upon the ability to begin to see the subtle drivers of how our patients come to care, and then tailor our team-approach treatment with that in mind. It is our mission to empower patients with information, perspective, and support; we want them always to know they have choices, including the choice of perspective and self-regulation in any stressful situation. Together we—my team, me, and especially my patients—can clearly pave the way for this to happen.

RESOURCES

Note: Many of the below resources are referenced solely to a website or websites current at the time of publication. They are of course subject to change. For those unable to access information in this manner, please feel free to contact me directly at the address below for further assistance.

Office Resources

Progressive-Dentistry, LLC
Jeffrey A. Oras, DMD
109 Main St., Whitehouse Station, NJ 08889
Office: (908) 534-5140
Fax: (908) 534-1921
www.progressive-dentistry.com
E-mail: jorasdmd@gmail.com

Kristen Belcastro
Reflexology & Reiki
Office: (908) 534-5140

Douglas Economy
Family Constellation
15 Southfield Dr.
PO Box 281
Pottersville, NJ 07979
Phone: (908) 343-8873
www.douglaseconomy.com
E-mail: info@douglaseconomy.com

Dr. Nancy Erb
Shifting Your Gears
N.E.T. (Neuro Emotional Technique)
EMDR (Eye Movement Desensitization Reprocessing)
1802 Rt. #31 North
Clinton, NJ 08809
Phone: (908) 268-0724
www.drnancyerb.com
E-mail: Dr_nancyerb@yahoo.com

United Angels Dream, LLC
Steven Cuoco—Re-connective Intuitive
Cell: (908) 329-5131
www.unitedangelsdream.com

Science Background Resources

Bowlby, John: *Attachment*

Bowlby, a British psychologist, psychiatrist, and psychoanalyst, and his research associate Mary Ainsworth are recognized as pioneers in the field of early childhood, especially for their development of now widely accepted attachment theory.

http://en.wikipedia.org/wiki/Attachment_theory

http://internal.psychology.illinois.edu/~rcfraley/attachment.htm

Klinghardt, Dietrich: Five Levels of Healing (Chart)

An integrative physician and teacher, Klinghardt's practice includes traditional and holistic components. He sees that healing takes place in realms other than the physical, and bases his treatment on referencing all of these realms, which he identifies as *physical, energy body, mental, intuitive,* and *spirit,* in ascending order of consciousness. I've included a link to a chart of these levels.

http://www.klinghardtacademy.com/5-Levels-of-Healing

Palmer, Brian: Importance of Breast-Feeding (Website Charts and Slideshow)

Palmer explores in detail the relation between breast-feeding and overall health.

http://www.brianpalmerdds.com/bfing_import.htm

Penfield, Wilder (Illustration)

Penfield was a Canadian neurosurgeon and teacher who devoted much thinking and research to the functionings of the mind.

http://en.wikipedia.org/wiki/Cortical_homunculus

Porges, Stephen: "The Polyvagal Theory: Phylogenetic Substrates of a Social Nervous System"

Porges is an educator and researcher responsible for developing a new model for the operation of the human autonomic system, which includes and explains the unique human phenomenon he identifies as the social engagement system.

http://en.wikipedia.org/wiki/Stephen_Porges

http://www.wisebrain.org/Polyvagal_Theory.pdf

Sato, Sadao and Rudolf Slavicek: "ATLAS Occlusion Diagnosis by BruxChecker" (Online Document)

These two researchers have proposed that teeth grinding (bruxism) is actually an excellent way to relieve stress.

http://www.kdcnet.ac.jp/college/occmed/pdf/atlasBruxChecker_e.pdf

Soesman, Albert: *Our Twelve Senses*

This is an extended explanation of noted educator and philosopher Rudolph Steiner's understanding of the influence of the operation of the human senses on quality of life. In this model, based on Steiner's postulations, twelve senses, rather than the usual five, are proposed: touch, life sense, self-movement, sense of balance, smell, taste, vision, temperature sense, hearing, speech or language sense, conceptual or idea sense, and ego sense.

http://www.amazon.com/Our-Twelve-Senses-Healthy-Refresh/dp/1869890752/ref=sr_1_2?s=books&ie=UTF8&qid=1341194140&sr=1-2&keywords=albert+soesman

Walker, Marsha (Website)

Walker is a prominent breast-feeding advocate, lactation consultant, and author of several useful books and monographs, identified in her website below.

http://www.ibreastfeeding.com/marsha-walker-rn-ibclc

Wilson, Ralph—Tooth-Organ Acumeridian Relationships (Website Charts)

The websites below contain much more extensive and detailed information than what is found on the chart found in the illustrations section of this book. Wilson synthesizes Western anatomy and physiology and the traditional Chinese meridian organs.

http://www.naturalworldhealing.com/Dentalinfo/toothorgan chart.htm

http://www.naturalconnectionshealthcare.com

Additional Science Resources

Davidson, Richard: *The Emotional Life of Your Brain*

Davidson suggests that our individual emotional responses are based upon how we respond or adapt within the following six dimensions: resilience, outlook, social intuition, self-awareness, sensitivity to context, and attention. He explores what he calls our individual "emotional style signature" and the premise that this signature is not rigidly embedded, but is subject to change in each of these dimensions. It provides a rich and detailed look at the emotional dimensions in how the brain receives, processes, and responds to input.

http://www.amazon.com/Emotional-Life-Your-Brain-Live--/dp/1594630895/ref=sr_1_1?s=books&ie=UTF8&qid=1341195 237&sr=1-1&keywords=the+emotional+life+of+your+brain+ric hard+davidson

Davidson, Terence: "The Great Leap Forward: The Anatomic Basis for the Acquisition of Speech and Obstructive Sleep Apnea"

This fascinating article posits the causes and effects of evolutionary changes in the human upper respiratory tract and identifies these changes as responsible for human loss of the epiglottis soft palate lock and the sleep disorder known as obstructive sleep apnea (OSA).

http://drdavidson.ucsd.edu/Portals/0/the%20great%20leap.pdf

Diamond, Jared: The Great Leap Forward (Website Monograph)

Diamond is an American scientist and author best known for his popular science books *The Third Chimpanzee; Guns, Germs, and Steel;* and *Collapse: How Societies Choose to Fail or Succeed.*

http://wps.pearsoncustom.com/wps/media/objects/6904/7070246/SOC250_Ch01.pdf

Gilbert, Dan: *Stumbling on Happiness*

Gilbert is a social psychologist known for his research on affective forecasting, with a special emphasis on cognitive biases, such as the impact bias. Gilbert's central thesis is that, through perception and cognitive biases, people imagine the future poorly, in particular what will make them happy. He examines the various ways that imagination fails in its ability to forecast future happiness or unhappiness.

http://en.wikipedia.org/wiki/Daniel_Gilbert_%28psychologist%29

http://www.amazon.com/Stumbling-Happiness-Daniel-Gilbert/dp/1400042666#reader_1400042666

Goleman, Daniel: *Emotional Intelligence*

Goleman is a prolific writer whose research into what makes for good leadership and decision making **has long been a standard reference in business schools as well as for anyone interested in broad insights about the effect of emotions on decision-making.**

http://danielgoleman.info/biography

http://www.amazon.com/Emotional-Intelligence-10th-Anniversary-Matter/dp/055380491X/ref=sr_1_1?s=books &ie=UTF8&qid=1341194975&sr=1-1&keywords=emotion al+intelligence+by+daniel+goleman

Gurian, Michael: What Could He Be Thinking? How a Man's Mind Really Works

Gurian points out here and in a number of other books what he considers nature-based, not culture-based, differences between men and women and explores how these biological and neurological differences shape behavior and relationships. Gurian suggests these differences thus have great impact on society as a whole. I am curious, though, to look further into the implications of his findings on my ability to fine-tune my support for patients based on gender.

http://www.amazon.com/exec/obidos/ASIN/0312311486/ qid=1069890789/sr=2-1/ref=sr_2_1/102-8811190-2660165

Roggenkamp, Clyde: Dentinal Fluid Transport

This little-known work describes and explains the research of Ralph Steinman, DDS, and John Leonora, DDS, into how hormonal function may determine the health or disease of a tooth.

http://www.amazon.com/Dentinal-Fluid-Transport-Clyde-Roggenkamp/dp/159410008X

Siegel, Dan: The Developing Mind, Second Edition: How Relationships and the Brain Interact to Shape Who We Are
Siegel's chief interest is the field of what he describes as interpersonal neurobiology. In this and other books, he investigates the way human relationships shape—and are shaped by—the brain, and the ways we may best assist the brain in accessing its inherently plastic aspects to change perspectives and promote human connection.
http://drdansiegel.com/

Siegel, Dan, and Marion Solomon: Healing Trauma: Attachment, Mind, Body, and Brain
This is another Siegel book, coauthored with a research colleague, Marion Solomon.
http://www.amazon.com/Healing-Trauma-Attachment-Mind-Brain/dp/0393703967

Acumeridian Tooth-Organ Relationships (Page 111)

Traditional Chinese Meridian Organs (Upper, Teeth 1–16)

Heart, Small Int., Circulation/Sex, Triple Warmer	Stomach, Pancreas	Lung, Large Intestine	Liver, Gallbladder	Kidney, Bladder	Kidney, Bladder	Liver, Gallbladder	Lung, Large Intestine	Stomach, Spleen	Heart, Small Int., Circulation/Sex, Triple Warmer

Associated Western Medicine Joints, Organs and Glands

- **Tooth 1** — Right: Shoulder, elbow, hand (ulnar). Sacroiliac, foot, toe. Middle Ear. Right heart. Rt. Duodenum, terminal Ileum. CNS. Ant pituitary
- **Tooth 2, 3** — Right: TMJ, anterior hip/knee, medial ankle. Sinus: Maxillary. Oropharynx. Larynx, esophagus. Rt. Side of Stomach. #3:Parathyroid; #2:Thyroid; Right Breast
- **Tooth 4, 5** — Right: Shoulder, elbow, hand (radial), foot, big toe. Sinus: Paranasal and Ethmoid. Bronchus, Nose. Right lung. Right side of Large Intestine. #4 Right Breast
- **Tooth 6** — Right: Post. knee, hip, lateral ankle. Sinus: Sphenoid. Palatine Tonsil. Eye. Right kidney, gallbladder.
- **Tooth 7, 8** — Right: Post. knee. Sacroiliac joint. Post. ankle. Sinus: Frontal. Pharyngeal Tonsil. Pineal. Right kidney, bladder, ovary, uterus, prostate, testicle, rectum
- **Tooth 9, 10** — Left: Post. knee. Sacroiliac joint. Post. ankle. Sinus: Frontal. Pharyngeal Tonsil. Pineal. Left kidney, bladder, ovary, uterus, prostate, testicle, rectum
- **Tooth 11** — Left: Post. knee, hip, lateral ankle. Sinus: Sphenoid. Palatine Tonsil. Eye. Left kidney, liver, biliary ducts.
- **Tooth 12, 13** — Left: Shoulder, elbow, hand (radial), foot, big toe. Sinus: Paranasal and Ethmoid. Bronchus, Nose. Left side of Large Intestine. #13 Left Breast
- **Tooth 14, 15** — Left: TMJ, anterior hip/knee, medial ankle. Sinus: Maxillary. Oropharynx. Larynx, esophagus. Left Side of Stomach. #15: Parathyroid; #14: Thyroid; Left Breast
- **Tooth 16** — Left: Shoulder, elbow, hand (ulnar). Sacroiliac, foot, toes. Middle Ear. Left heart. Jejunum, Ileum. CNS. Ant pituitary

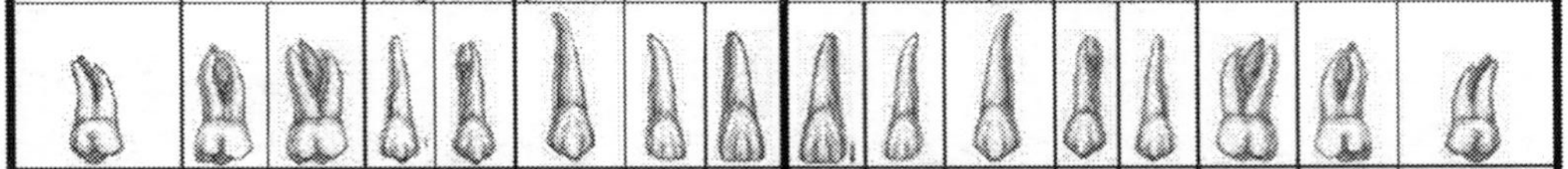

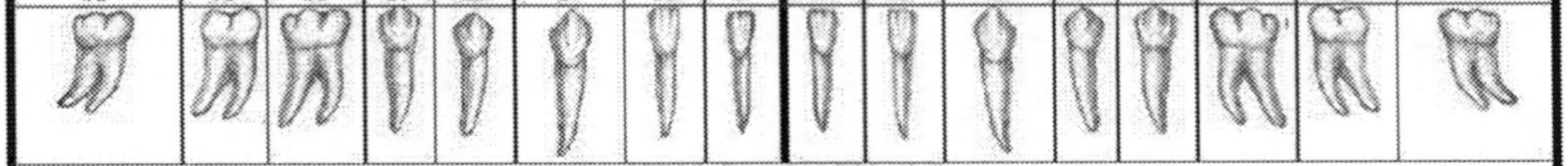

Teeth numbered 1–16 (top row) and 32–17 (lower row).

Traditional Chinese Meridian Organs (Lower, Teeth 17–32)

Heart, Small Int., Circulation/Sex, Triple Warmer	Lung, Large Intestine	Stomach, Pancreas	Liver, Gallbladder	Kidney, Bladder	Kidney, Bladder	Liver, Gallbladder	Spleen, Stomach	Lung, Large Intestine	Heart, Small Int., Circulation/Sex, Triple Warmer

Associated Western Medicine Joints, Organs and Glands

- Right: Shoulder, elbow, hand (ulnar). Sacroiliac, foot, toes. Middle Ear. Right heart. Rt. Duodenum, terminal Ileum. CNS.
- Right: Shoulder, elbow, hand (radial). Sinus: Paranasal and Ethmoid. Bronchus, Nose. Right lung. Right side of Large Intestine.
- Right: TMJ, anterior hip/knee. Sinus: Maxillary. Oropharynx. Larynx, esophagus. Rt. Side of Stomach. #29 Ovaries; Testes. Right Breast
- Right: Post. knee, hip, lateral ankle. Sinus: Sphenoid. Palatine Tonsil. Eye. Rt. Liver, gallbladder.
- Right: Post. knee. Sacroiliac joint. Post. ankle. Sinus: Frontal. Pharyngeal Tonsil. Adrenal. Right kidney, bladder, ovary, uterus, prostate, testicle, rectum
- Left: Post. knee. Sacroiliac joint. Post. ankle. Sinus: Frontal. Pharyngeal Tonsil. Adrenal. Left kidney, bladder, ovary, uterus, prostate, testicle, rectum
- Left: Post. knee, hip, lateral ankle. Sinus: Sphenoid. Palatine Tonsil. Eye. Left. Liver, biliary ducts.
- Left: TMJ, anterior hip/knee, medial ankle. Sinus: Maxillary. Oropharynx. Larynx, esophagus. Left Side of Stomach. #21; Ovaries; Testes. Left Breast
- Left: Shoulder, elbow, hand (radial), foot, big toe. Sinus: Paranasal and Ethmoid. Bronchus, Nose. Left lung. Left side Large Intestine
- Left: Shoulder, elbow, hand (ulnar). Sacroiliac, foot, toes. Middle Ear. Left heart. Jejunum, Ileum. CNS. Ant pituitary

Acumeridian Tooth-Organ Relationships from various sources including Gleditsch and Klinghardt (www.NeuralTherapy.com). Compiled by: Dr. Ralph Wilson

Jeffrey A. Oras, DMD, is currently an actively practicing dentist in Whitehouse Station, New Jersey. A graduate of Fairleigh Dickinson University School of Dentistry, he and his wife live in Lebanon, New Jersey.